Practicing Thomas Szasz

Continuing the Work of the Philosopher of Liberty

I0117982

John Breeding, PhD

chipmunkapublishing
the mental health publisher

John Breeding, PhD

Published by
Chipmunkapublishing
United Kingdom

http://www.chipmunkapublishing.com

Copyright © 2014 John Breeding, PhD

ISBN   978-1-78382-132-7

Chipmunkapublishing gratefully acknowledge the support of Arts Council England.

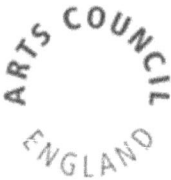

Dedication

John Friedberg was a good friend and admirer of Tom Szasz, and he died on May 19, 2012, shortly before Szasz. Friedberg was a long-time California neurologist, and an activist against psychiatric oppression, and especially against electroshock. He wrote the book, *Shock Treatment Is Not Good for Your Brain*, in 1978, and remained active—I testified with him before state legislative committees in Texas and in New York, where shock was being challenged. Friedberg liked to tell the story of how, as a newly minted physician in search of a medical specialty, he was drawn to psychiatry, and went to personally consult with Szasz about his decision. Szasz warned him against psychiatry, pointing out the virtual impossibility of an ethical practice. John chose neurology, and became one of the persons through whom Szasz influenced me and others as well.

To Thomas Szasz: born April 15, 1920; died September 8, 2012.

John Breeding, PhD

Table of Contents

John Breeding, PhD

Introduction

Thomas Szasz died at 92 on September 8, 2012. With his death, many of us, not enough, are left with deep concern about his legacy and the continuing influence of his ideas. Here, following a biographical sketch, I discuss some of the myriad ways his ideas have directly or indirectly influenced my ongoing work as a psychologist. I hope that my experience will have a small positive effect in keeping alive and in play the profoundly important ideas of this great man.

Szasz became a psychiatrist with the thought of launching an attack on psychiatry that would end or at least significantly reduce the use of civil commitment and the insanity defense. He stayed true to this goal throughout his life. At the same time, he would not advise another to follow in his footsteps. Nevertheless, he has educated and inspired me, hence the focus of this book is on how his work influences my own.

I have been involved in the so-called mental health field for about 40 years. My first job after graduating from college with a bachelor's degree in psychology in 1975 was in a residential treatment center for children. During my three years there I learned about the systematic drugging of children, which even then was not uncommon. Like Szasz in his choice of a residency in psychiatry, I went on to study psychology in graduate school because I wanted to work with people. I knew that there were problems with the profession I was entering, that people in the field were engaged in unethical, harmful practices, but was not nearly as clear as Szasz in my understanding of the profession; nor did I have, like him, an agenda to completely expose and preferably destroy coercive psychiatry.

I barely knew about Szasz at the time. I had heard of *The Myth of Mental Illness*, and when I finally read that classic, I understood the main point, but got bogged down in his game theory analysis of human behavior and lost interest. As a child of the '60s, I gravitated to the work of the British psychiatrist R.D. Laing—a man Szasz abhorred (Szasz, 2008a)—and read many of his books. Laing's writing was helpful in offering a radical criticism of standard psychiatric ideology and practice, especially as a fresh buffer and counterweight to the mainstream teachings of the schools I attended. So by the time I became a psychologist in 1983, I knew enough to be concerned about my profession. I think I had the idea, however, that I could be a counselor, reject the medical model of "mental illness," and somehow separate myself from the dehumanization that Laing wrote about.

Early on as a counselor, that fantasy died. As client after client came in already hurt by prior experiences at the hands of my fellow "mental health professionals," the profound question of how to be ethical in a largely unethical profession gained a harsh immediacy. It became clear that the only way to remain in my profession would be to focus my activist energies, which to that point had mostly been on peace and justice issues, on becoming a dissident psychologist. It seemed to me that even my progressive allies had a huge blind spot when it came to psychiatric oppression, so I thought I might serve as a bridge between the general progressive movement and the folks who I thought of as members of the mental health liberation movement. In any event, like Szasz when he chose a psychiatric residency, I now I had an agenda. By reading dissident psychiatrist Peter Breggin's *Toxic Psychiatry* (1991), I learned more about the harmfulness of psychiatry's biological "treatments," but it was Szasz who became my main teacher regarding the application of ethics in my work as a psychologist.

In general, my study of Szasz has allowed me to imbibe much of his vision, and thus cut through the mystification and obfuscation that passes as psychiatric theory and practice today. In this book, I will describe and give examples of some of Szasz's principles that have shaped and continue to influence my work. That influence comes primarily from his writings, but also indirectly through the influence on me of several of his followers.

The core of Szasz' work is about liberty and responsibility. Part I of this book is a biographical essay, originally published in a slightly different form in the *Journal of Humanistic Psychology* (Breeding, 2011), that provides a window into this great man's life. The heart of the book, parts II-IV, is about Szasz's continuing influence on my own work. I try to share what it looks like, in my own experience, to "practice Szasz" as a mental health professional. Specific areas that I discuss include issues of power and coercion, and psychiatry and the law. I also consider deeper and subtler influences regarding language, as well as the effect of Szasz as a model of precision, determination and courage. Finally, given that I am a professional counselor, and that Szasz worked for decades as a counselor, I discuss his ideas about counseling per se, and how they have affected my own work. A final, special gift is the appendix of select quotations offering a small feast of the ideas of the brilliant Thomas Szasz in his own words, edited by Leonard Roy Frank.

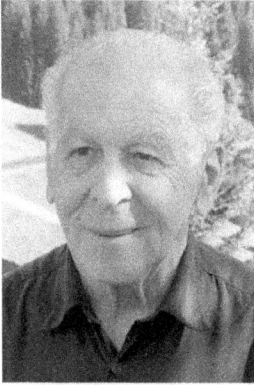 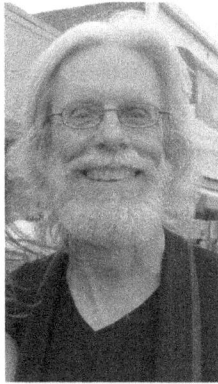

Thomas Szasz   John Breeding

John Breeding, PhD

Part I

THOMAS SZASZ: PHILOSOPHER OF LIBERTY
(A Biographical Sketch)

John Breeding, PhD

THOMAS SZASZ: PHILOSOPHER OF LIBERTY

To make good the cause of Freedom against Slavery
you must be...
Declarations of Independence walking.
—Ralph Waldo Emerson, "Notebook WO Liberty" (1855, p. 199)

It is a rare and precious gift to be writing about Thomas Szasz, who turned 90 on April 15, 2010—a living sage whose mind is sharper than my own and whose mental energy and productivity is astounding. In this coming year, we saw the 50th anniversary edition of his book that marked his full-scale assault on coercive psychiatry—*The Myth of Mental Illness*. In the past 4 years, he has added dozens of articles and a handful of major books to his incredible body of work (see http://www.szasz.com).

One of the enduring sayings of a great rabbi teacher, the man called Jesus, is that, "By their fruits you will know them" (Matthew 7:20 NKJV). As a philosopher, however, Szasz's primary mission is not to convey words, but wisdom. The prime fruit of that tree are those who grow and deepen their understanding as a result of partaking in his ideas. My friend, Leonard Roy Frank, author and relentless activist in the movement for liberation from psychiatric oppression, is a prime example. More than anyone, Frank helped me, to borrow the words of Bob Marley, "decolonize my mind" by systematically examining and challenging my use of language as a "mental health" professional. I know with greater certainty, for example, that "civil commitment" really means incarceration and that forced "treatment" generally means assault with a potentially deadly weapon—and I know how important it is to say it that way. Frank cut some serious teeth in this domain by reading Szasz, so the master's direct influence on my thinking has at least been matched by his indirect influence via Frank and others.

Though Szasz's critics may see people like Frank and myself as poisoned fruit, the fact is we are most definitely clearer and stronger by virtue of our relationship with Szasz. So are countless other students of his work, including, for example, neurologist John Friedberg and psychologists Seth Farber and Jeff Rubin.

Although Szasz has been prolific in the dissemination of his ideas, much less has been known about his personal history and psychology. It was striking, as I read more about Szasz as seen by his colleagues, how little had been revealed about the man.. For example, the first really intensive examination of Szasz and his works was initiated by Keith Hoeller, and became a special issue of the *Review of Existential Psychology and Psychiatry* (1997). As Hoeller (1997) wrote in his "Editor's Introduction," "When I called Thomas Szasz to offer to edit a Festschrift in his honor, I fully expected to hear from him that several either had already been done, which I had somehow overlooked, or that several were underway.... I was frankly surprised such was not the case...." (p. 1). To this day there is still no book-length biography. There is, however, one thing almost as good—Szasz's own 28-page autobiographical sketch, published in the book edited by psychologist Jeffrey A. Schaler, *Szasz Under Fire* (2004).

Szasz Tamas Istvan was born in Budapest, Hungary on April 15, 1920. Family and friends called him Tomi, similar to the English "Tom," by which he is still known to his current friends. Born into an upper-class family, Szasz's primary caregiver during his first 10 years was his beloved governess, Kisu. After age 10, he spent much more time with his parents, whom he deeply loved and respected. The close lifelong relationship with older brother George, whom Szasz asserts is much smarter than himself, has been an essential fact and joy of his existence.

There are some fascinating jewels for the biographically inclined in Szasz's brief personal sketch. For example, Szasz had many childhood illnesses, including chicken pox, whooping cough, measles, scarlet fever, and diphtheria! As a young boy he learned to malinger because he much preferred staying home to school: "My illnesses taught me some valuable lessons. One was a clear realization of the advantages of being ill.... I learned to malinger....how to have a fever.... by surreptitiously placing the thermometer close to a lighted light bulb (Szasz, 2004a, p. 4). Despite Szasz's aforementioned resolve to keep his personal and professional lives separate, it is intriguing to "analyze" this history in light of Szasz's early works on strategic interaction and the role of malingering in psychiatric diagnosis; but that is speculation. An important fact is that he was largely self-taught: "I always preferred to learn, rather than be taught" (2004a, p. 21). With the aid of books he became his own teacher. His autobiography provides sure evidence of a family and school culture that emphasized scholarship and critical thinking, both of which Szasz came to excel in.

Szasz learned from his family the virtues of respectfulness, cordiality, and consideration. While his opponents obviously do not agree, my experience is that he is unfailingly expresses these qualities in his writings, talks, and conversations. At age 84, he wrote, "Politeness: one of the most neglected and underrated virtues of our age" Szasz, 2004b). Szasz also places great value on being direct and honest. He is often intensely confrontational in his writings; witness, for example, his scathing criticism of R.D. Laing (2008). Some (e.g., Burston, 2003) think Szasz is overly harsh on his opponents.

Szasz says he also "inherited" the traits of being well-groomed and well-dressed! He kept a full range of friends at each stage of his life. As a youngster, he stoked his competitive athletic fires in intense pingpong with George, and remained active in sports, primarily tennis, throughout most of life. At the young age of 18, he emigrated to the United States and landed in Cincinnati where his uncle, a renowned professor of mathematics, taught at the University of Cincinnati. He came to this country knowing but few words and phrases in English, but three years later, in 1941, he graduated from the University of Cincinnati with honors in physics. We get glimpses of other nonacademic lessons for this young man, for example, refusal of a restaurant to allow him to sit and eat with a friend who happened to be an Afro-American (Szasz, 2004a, p. 14). During his last year as an undergraduate, Szasz applied to 26 medical schools but was systematically rejected one after another as "undesirable" when, despite thinking of himself as an atheist, he affirmed his Jewish heritage. Probably because people knew him and his esteemed uncle, (2004a, p. 15), he was admitted to the University of Cincinnati College of Medicine and graduated in 1944, first in his class.

These examples of Szasz's awareness and sensitivity to the various faces of oppression—racism and anti-Semitism—enable us to better understand his motivation to become a freedom fighter. Obviously best known for his work in challenging psychiatric oppression, Szasz has never failed to place this challenge in a large context. He is a master of aphorism and analogy, and my own favorite summarizes his classic, *The Manufacture of Madness: A Comparative Study of the Inquisition and the Mental Health Movement* (Szasz, 1970):

> The Inquisition is to heresy as Psychiatry is to mental illness.

Szasz has sensitized generations of citizens to the fact that psychiatry is first and foremost an agent of social control. The title

of another of his books, *Liberation by Oppression: A Comparative Study of Slavery and Psychiatry* (Szasz, 2002), is in a similar vein. Both books starkly reveal a fundamental teaching of oppression theory, that all oppression is justified by claims to virtue.
Szasz has done heroic, masterful work in laying bare the moral bankruptcy of such claims. When he speaks of psychiatric slavery, he is in a long line of liberation workers who refuse to silence victims with the oppressors' twisted logic and the phoney claims to virtue. Szasz is expressing compassion and zeal for freedom when he shares the voices of those citizens who protest their involuntary "commitment and treatment" which they regard as imprisonment and torture.

A self-described primary compelling force in Szasz's life has been curiosity, as he phrased it, to "know what's under the hood." He did an unpaid apprenticeship in an auto repair garage before leaving Europe and learned how to drive, so that when he came to the United States he was the only member of his family who could drive! In an astounding example of investment of energy, once he finished all his medical training, he walked away from medicine as he had gotten what he wanted—a better understanding of what was under the hood of the human body. Later, Szasz practiced medicine for two years in the Navy, from 1954 to 1956. Szasz does indeed have a deep and abiding curiosity:

> Although I have an abiding interest in and love for medicine and the hard sciences, my true passion was literature, history, philosophy, politics—or, put more plainly, how and why people live, suffer and die. (2004a, p. 17)

> Strange as it may sound, just as I wanted to go to medical school to learn medicine, not to practice it, I served a psychiatric residency to qualify as a psychiatrist and be eligible for training in psychoanalysis, not to practice psychiatry. I felt that I would rather earn a living as a psychoanalyst than as an internist; that I would then have more leisure and opportunity to pursue my intellectual—literary, social, political— interests, and that the role of psychoanalyst would provide a platform from which *I could perhaps launch an attack on what I had long felt were the immoral practices of civil commitment and the insanity defense* [italics added]. (2004a, p. 18)

I want to emphasize the two reasons Szasz did a psychiatric residency— he wanted to train as a psychoanalyst and he needed a platform for a specific agenda. First, the training.

Szasz has written so much, and there are so many misconceptions deliberate or otherwise—about his work that it has felt overwhelming to choose what to write about. As a professional psychologist, it has been gratifying to learn by more closely studying his life that he is a brother not only in the work of challenging psychiatric oppression but also in the work of professional counseling. It is easy to miss this, partly because of Szasz's felt imperative to focus on the very main challenge of his work, which is to defend liberty and destroy tyranny in his chosen profession. Even more of a blinder is that this part of Szasz's life gets so twisted and distorted by his critics who decry him as a cold, uncaring "right-wing nut" who would prefer to deny people's "mental illness" and let them suffer rather than help them. Reading both the historical and the current criticisms of Szasz, this type of *ad hominem* attack is relentless. Also relentless is the straw-man argument that those of us who reject psychiatric coercion and the fraudulent declaration of theory as fact simply want to let people suffer and die, and offer nothing. In his response to the belittlement of Ralph Slovenko (2004), professor of psychiatry and law at Wayne State University, in *Szasz Under Fire*, Szasz writes, "The point is that Slovenko disapproves of the way I practiced 'listening and talking' for some fifty years . . ." (2004e, p. 162). Thomas Szasz not only trained as a psychoanalyst, he worked *for some fifty years* as a counselor.

Some critics argue that Szasz's constant reference to the Virchowian gold standard of physical or chemical abnormality as the only valid criteria of disease leaves him defending an untenable belief in the face of decades of research that renders obsolete the old, absolute distinction between mind and body. Daniel Burston (2003), for example, changes Szasz's famous aphorism, "mental illness is a myth," to "mental illness is not a myth, but an oxymoron," since psychological suffering very often also entails bodily suffering. These are important points for the field of counseling, but in my mind at least they are secondary to the main work of Szasz, which is about coercion and responsibility. They also beg the tragic fact that alleged biological (chemical imbalance theory) and genetic (bad gene theory) defects are used to justify a whole range of brain-disabling "treatment" with drugs and electroshock.

I think that part of Szasz's intense effort to disabuse people of the notion that he is an antipsychiatrist (Szasz, 2008) is to remind us that he is a psychiatrist and not against himself. He is against coercion as civil commitment and excuse-making as the insanity defense. He will engage folks on the validity of the "mental illness" metaphor, but he would defend forever their right to believe what they wish. He would and does also defend the right of all citizens, including those called "mentally ill," to be free from coercion; and he has and does insist on accountability for those who commit crimes.

Burston also discusses the issue of confidentiality and represents those who see things in a much grayer way than does Szasz who holds confidentiality as a sacrosanct part of the counselor–client contract. Burston argues that Szasz's constant framing of things as adversarial as in state versus "patient" and family versus "patient" creates a sometimes false and sometimes even harmful divisiveness. Burston concludes that for counselors, "confidentiality has limits"; he sees this position as a greater valuing of life than confidentiality. One can easily imagine Szasz's response to this. Burston is thoughtful enough to at least admit his resulting conundrum. Even though he espouses agreement with Szasz's fundamental rejection of coercion, he is willing to risk that those with whom he might choose to violate confidentiality might not share that rejection; "if so, that cannot be helped" (p. 5).

Burston, who wrote a book about R.D. Laing, takes issue with Szasz's harsh assessment of him. He also argues that Laing's personal failings, albeit severe, should not deter one from evaluating his ideas on their own merits. I would say two things about this. One, my embrace of Szasz's fundamental teachings related to psychiatric oppression as a form of state and social control disguised as medicine certainly does not require agreement with all his ideas and attitudes. My second point is expressed in the following quote attributed to Lord Acton, that I found in *Szasz Under Fire* (2004d) . It remedies some of the confusion related to the contentious issues engaged by Szasz and his critics:

> To renounce the pains and penalties of exhaustive research is to remain a victim of ill-informed and designing writers, and to authorities that have worked for ages to build up the vast tradition of conventional mendacity." (p. 223)

In a December 2000 interview, Szasz told Randall Wyatt that he found doing therapy quite satisfying, but that one of the reasons he left Chicago for Syracuse was to escape having to support himself financially by doing therapy because that can create financial temptations to make clients dependent on therapy. He also shared the following with Wyatt:

> When practicing psychiatry—psychotherapy—I never prescribed a drug. I never gave insulin shock or electric shock. I never committed anyone. I never testified in court that a criminal was not responsible for his crimes. I never saw, as a patient, anyone who did not want to see me.
> I went into psychiatry with my eyes wide open. I never viewed psychiatry or psychotherapy as a part of medicine. Perhaps I should add, though it should be obvious, that I had no objections to the patient taking drugs or doing anything else he wanted. As far as I was concerned, things outside the consulting room were not my business—in the sense that if the patient wanted to take drugs, he had to go to a doctor and get them, just as if he wanted a divorce, he had to go to a lawyer.

Szasz practiced counseling, but as acknowledged earlier he was also indeed "treacherous." Not only did he have a greater affinity with the humanistic psychologists, for example, than with his fellow psychiatrists, he overtly supported all the nonmedical counselors over the guild interests of psychiatry that wanted to assert its supreme value as purveyor of "mental health treatment." During the years before "medical" psychiatry won out, Szasz continually asserted that counseling was not a medical issue, but a conversation between people. It is understandable that psychiatrists felt betrayed; in a sense they were. Szasz's allegiance was not to his guild, but to the truth. The reactions of Slovenko and other critics is a mostly blind aggression in defense of their "right" to imprison and poison (or electrocute) citizens without due process of law, in the name of medicine. Of course, the essential point is that because "mental illness" is not a disease there can be no treatment for it.

Szasz had begun a medical residency in Cincinnati in July of 1945, and within a few months, decided "to bite the proverbial bullet." He would complete this residency in internal medicine, through March of 1946, then quit medicine. He told the chairman of the department that he was going to apply for a residency in psychiatry. The chair responded by telling Szasz that "Medicine is losing a good man," thus affirming Szasz's major theme that psychiatry is not a part of medicine (2004a, p. 18).

Szasz went to Chicago for a psychiatry residency because it emphasized psychoanalysis and was loosely structured. "The residency at the University of Chicago was ideal for me, not least because no one made any attempt to teach me anything. I always preferred to learn, rather than be taught. I read widely, had many intelligent friends, played bridge and tennis regularly, and read a lot" (Szasz, 2004a, p. 21). However, he writes, "this idyll came to an abrupt end," in the form of a replacement of the department chair by "a freshly demobilized psychiatrist" (p. 21), Henry Brosin. According to Szasz the two got along very well, and often played tennis as they were evenly matched. But one day, "Brosin called me into his office for a chat." Basically, Brosin decided that the Chicago residency needed to provide "experience with treating seriously ill patients." This meant that Szasz would be required to do his third year of residency at Cook County Hospital. Szasz told Brosin that he preferred to stay where he was.

> I was not about to tell him that the persons he called "seriously ill patients" I regarded as persons deprived of liberty by psychiatrist. I still felt much too vulnerable to let my superiors, or even friends, know what I thought about mental illnesses and psychiatric coercion. After a moment's hesitation, I thanked him, and said, "Hank, I tell you what, I quit". . . I did not tell Brosin that ever since I was an adolescent, when I set my sights on going to medical school, I had believed that the physician's role is to help relieve the suffering of individuals who ask for and accept his help, and that the psychiatrist is committing a grave moral wrong if he imprisons individuals who neither seek nor want his help. (Szasz, 2004a, p. 21)

Fortunately, Szasz was well-liked and well-respected and found much more suitable ways to complete his training in Chicago. Those were exciting years for him:

> Everything I had learned and thought about mental illness, psychiatry, and psychoanalysis—from my teenage years through medical school, and my psychiatric and psychoanalytic training—confirmed my view that mental illness is a fiction; that psychiatry, resting on force and fraud is social control; and that psychoanalysis—properly conceived— has nothing to do with illness or medicine or treatment, but is a special kind of confidential dialogue that often helps people resolve some of their personal

problems and may help them improve their ability to cope with the slings and arrows of outrageous fortune.

Still, I had to keep my beliefs—or, better, disbeliefs—to myself. I was poor, I was in debt, I had to earn a living. It was obvious that my view of psychoanalysis, as an enterprise separate from psychiatry—indeed, conceptually, economically, and morally antithetical to it— was not shared by my teachers or fellow trainees. (Szasz, 2004a, p. 22)

Szasz's autobiographical sketch deliberately leaves off just as he moved, with his wife and two young daughters, to Syracuse in 1956, at age 36, to assume a position as tenured professor of psychiatry. He could support his family, and he was tenured—fair protection against certain professional and political vulnerabilities. And he has vigorously wielded his intellectual sword ever since. Syracuse is where he began in earnest the work that made him famous—a work that is, by all accounts, favorable or not, an intellectual tour de force. Syracuse is the place where Szasz launched an epic, sustained campaign against his chosen profession. He himself acknowledges 1956 "as the year that my treachery began" (2004e, p. 175).

Beyond psychoanalysis per se, Szasz's other agenda in choosing a psychiatric residency is directly relevant to his subsequent notoriety within the psychiatric profession, as well as his relative obscurity without. The fundamental, irreconcilable conflict between those who choose to value paternalistic coercion, in the flimsy guise of pseudoscientifc medicine, on the one hand, and those who would defend liberty, autonomy and self-determination, on the other, is the heart of Szasz's life work. This work is how I and many others connected with the man. I was an activist challenging the many faces of militarism before I became a "mental health professional" and more deeply confronted the exceedingly difficult, though very common dilemma of how to be ethical in a largely unethical profession. As revealed above, Szasz did a psychiatric residency with a specific, *destructive* intention toward his chosen profession! I was a bit slower on the uptake and was fortunate to have Szasz to help me understand what I was facing every day with the clients I loved and respected. He helped me reach a vital clarity that allows me to counsel people without being oppressive, and to actively challenge psychiatric oppression in the world. This clarity includes, of course, understanding that psychiatry's twin pillars—involuntary commitment and the insanity defense—are an assault on freedom.

It also includes clarity about the rhetoric of suicide (Szasz, 1999) that so frequently turns a counselor into an agent of the state in incarcerating and forcibly "treating" innocent people. Beyond the specifics, reading or listening to Szasz is one of the best techniques for enhancing one's ability to think clearly—period.

It is interesting to read some of Szasz's critics in *Szasz Under Fire*, who suggest that he failed in his effort to destroy psychiatry because he was too extreme, that he should have settled for challenging the excesses, the abuses in psychiatry. In his response to one of these men, Edinburgh psychiatrist Robert Kendall, Szasz once again asserts that he never intended to reform psychiatry. He long ago concluded that, given the unholy symbiotic twinship between the force of state law and psychiatry, reform was impossible—one of the twins had to die. Since the power of the state was not going away, that left psychiatry. In his reply to Kendell, Szasz (2004c) stated that "I consider being able to articulate that viewpoint—and attracting a hearing for it—as much success as I ever hoped for" (p. 53).

Henry Weihofen, a leading forensic psychiatrist at the time, denounced Szasz, in 1964, as a heartless fascist and "extremist right winger." Szasz says, "Since then, virtually all defenders of psychiatric slavery have leveled this charge against me" (2004e, p. 178).

In the aforementioned 2000 interview, Wyatt asked Szasz how he dealt with the relentless criticism:

> I was very fortunate. I had very good parents, a very good brother, a very good education as a child in Budapest. I have very fine children, good friends, good health, good habits, a fair amount of intelligence.
> Really, I have always felt blessed. It also helped at lot that I felt there were many people who agreed with me—that what I'm simply saying is simply 2 + 2 = 4—but that many people are afraid to say this when it is personally and politically improvident to do so. I haven't made any scientific discoveries. I'm simply saying that if you are white and don't like blacks, or vice versa, that's not a disease, it's a prejudice. If you're in a building that you can't get out of, that's not a hospital, it's a prison.
> I don't care how many people call racism an illness or involuntary mental hospitalization a treatment.

Szasz did acknowledge that the criticism concerned him at times, especially when people actually wanted to injure me—personally, professionally, legally.... I tried to protect myself and escaped, luckily enough. I found boundless support in literature, in the great writers.Ibsen said, among other things, that "the compact majority is always wrong."

Wyatt asked Szasz about his heroes:

> Where should I start, there are many? Shakespeare, Goethe, Adam Smith, Jefferson, Madison, John Stuart Mill, Mark Twain, Mencken. Tolstoy, Dostoyevski, Chekhov. Orwell, C.S. Lewis. Ludwig von Mises, F. A. Hayek, Camus, and Sartre, though personally and politically, he is rather despicable. He was a Communist sympathizer. He was willing to overlook the Gulag. But he was very insightful into the human condition. His autobiography is superb. His book on anti- Semitism is important.

As in the general case of seeking truth, the simplistic dichotomy of left and right is useless in understanding Szasz. Over and again, Szasz has shown his affinity with liberal humanists such as Thomas Jefferson and John Stuart Mill, Adam Smith and Lord Acton. I learned a Josh Billings quote awhile back from Szasz, that "The problem is not that people don't know anything, but that they know so many things that ain't so." Szasz has been perhaps my best help over the years in clearing or defending against the effects of the constant drumbeat of psychiatric propaganda. Regarding his political leanings: "For me the issue is, and has always been, individualism versus statism, not "right-wing" or "left-wing" (Szasz, 2004e, p. 176).

The historian Howard Zinn—a man who might be categorized as being on the far "left"—once commented on how presidents, both Democratic and Republican, always lie to get the country to go to war: "If you don't know history, it is as if you were born yesterday." Time and again, Szasz emphasizes the importance of knowing history and does the work of forcing the history of psychiatry into the public eye. I did a video review of one of my personal favorites, his history book, *Coercion as Cure: A Critical History of Psychiatry* (Breeding, 2009).

While it is true that today overt slavery and racism at least tend to be frowned upon, Szasz believes that psychiatry replaced the

Inquisition and snuffed out whatever "enlightenment" there was following the latter's quiet demise. In any event, one technique that buttresses the claims to virtue is to rewrite or simply "forget" history. This is why Szasz has so painstakingly and repeatedly unearthed and exposed the history of psychiatry. In challenging electroshock, Leonard Frank's *Electroshock Quotationary* (2008) is the best source for the truth about electroshock's history, including the fact that the early shock doctors applauded brain damage, the procedure's primary and most obvious effect. I mention this here because I found the following ironic quote from Hungarian-born psychiatrist Paul Hoch in Frank's book:

> This brings us for a moment to a discussion of the brain damage produced by electroshock . . . Is a certain amount of brain damage not necessary in this type of treatment? Frontal lobotomy indicates that improvement takes place by a definite damage of certain parts of the brain. (Paul H. Hoch, "Discussion and Concluding Remarks," *Journal of Personality*, vol. 17, 1948)

Paul Hoch is the man who, in his position as commissioner of the New York State Department of Mental Hygiene, insisted on the firing of Thomas Szasz from his teaching position at Syracuse Psychiatric Hospital in 1962 (Hoch,1962/2004).

A more general—and more seminal to the underground history of psychiatry—statement providing an accurate rationale for psychiatric coercion and assault belongs to Benjamin Rush, the "founding father" of American psychiatry, a man whose profile emblazons the seal of the American Psychiatric Association:

> TERROR acts powerfully upon the body, through the medium of the mind, and should be employed in the cure of madness.... FEAR, accompanied with PAIN, and a sense of SHAME, has sometimes cured this disease. Bartholin speaks in high terms of what he calls "flagellation" in certain diseases. (Benjamin Rush, *Medical Inquiries and Observations, Upon the Diseases of the Mind*, chap. 7, 1812)

The work of unearthing history is important for any domain where truth and understanding is desired. To my mind, the work of John Taylor Gatto lends perspective to the stupid notion that Szasz, and all his allies, failed to stop the sickening wave and horrific effects of what one lawyer calls "the pharmacaust" because of faulty ideas or strategy. Like Szasz a Libertarian, Gatto is a lifelong teacher, but he quit the public schools with a bang on January 31, 1990 when, on the occasion of accepting an award from the New York State Senate naming him New York City Teacher of the Year he gave his celebrated—at least in alternative education circles—speech, "The Psychopathic School."

Gatto (2000) also wrote a history book, *The Underground History of Modern Education*, in which he details his extensive research into the designs of those who planned and implemented our modern system of compulsory public education, the keyword in any essay about Szasz being, of course, compulsory! Here is a piece of Gatto's research, a quote from William Torrey Harris, U.S. Commissioner of Education from 1889 to 1906, who, according to Gatto, played the key role in standardizing our schools, according to the Prussian (German) model:

> Ninety-nine [students] out of a hundred are automata, careful to walk in prescribed paths, careful to follow the prescribed custom. This is not an accident but the result of substantial education, which, scientifically defined, is the subsumption of the individual. (The Philosophy of Education, 1906; cited in Gatto, p. 106)

Szasz knew the dangers of Harris's assertion early on:

> I realized, even before I left Hungary, that psychiatrists and psychoanalysis had nothing to do with real medicine or with one another: psychiatrists locked up troublesome persons in insane asylums for the benefit of their relatives; psychoanalysts, who were not supposed to touch their patients, engaged in a particular kind of conversation with them. Incarcerating people and talking to them were not medicine. Any intelligent child would have known that. Of course, such simpleminded clarity had to be "educated" out of people to make them normal members of society, especially American society. (Szasz, 2004a, pp. 17-18)

In his autobiographical essay, Szasz says that he was deeply moved by the tragic story of Hungarian obstetrician Ignaz Semmelweis. Semmelweis has been called the "savior of mothers" for his discovery that childbed fever, a form of septicemia, could be prevented if doctors washed their hands in a chlorine solution before gynecological exams. During his life, however, the medical profession angrily challenged and denounced them. Subsequently, according to Wikipedia (2010),

> His contemporaries, including his wife, believed he was losing his mind, and in 1865 he was committed to an asylum. In an ironic twist of fate, he died there of septicaemia only 14 days later, possibly after being severely beaten by guards.

It was only after his death, with the discoveries of Louis Pasteur, that his ideasgained widespread acceptance. Here is what young Szasz learned from Semmelweis's story:

> It taught me, at an early age, the lesson that it can be dangerous to be wrong, but, to be right, when society regards the majority's falsehood as truth, could be fatal. This principle is especially true with respect to false truths that form an important part of society's belief system. (Szasz, 2004a, p. 27)

Szasz has not had to pay with his life, but he has paid dearly— attacked, criticized, dismissed, and censored. When "all hell broke loose" at Syracuse shortly after the publication of *The Myth of Mental Illness* and public testimony at a well-publicized commitment hearing, Szasz was fired from a position at the allied state hospital; they were not able to fire him from his tenured professorship, but tried to make him pay in other ways. One of the hardest things must have been to see his close friends and colleagues who supported him be systematically purged from the department and retaliated against beyond that.

One of the men who was purged from Syracuse, psychiatrist Ron Leifer, wrote a summary of that experience for the aforementioned *Review of Existential Psychology and Psychiatry* tribute to Szasz, titled, "The Psychiatric Repression of Dr. Thomas Szasz: Its Social and Political Significance." The very close alliance of the Syracuse psychiatry department with the New York State Department of Mental Hygiene (DMH) presented a severe ethical conflict of interest, epitomized by the fact that the department head, Marc Hollender, was also director of Syracuse Psychiatric (State) Hospital. Many other faculty had joint appointments, a common arrangement then and now.

This is why DMH director, Paul Hoch (quoted above regarding his views on the value of brain damage in psychiatric treatment) could in 1962 order Hollender to "terminate Dr. Szasz" to prevent his having contact with the residents of the state institutions and any personnel who are employed by the Department of Mental Hygiene (Hoch, 1962/2004).

When Hollender suggested Szasz move his seminars for the psychiatric residents to the University, Szasz refused this compromise—he and his allies, people like Ron Leifer and Pulitzer Prize winner Ernest Becker, fought hard for academic freedom. They strongly believed that this example of repression dramatically underscored the principle that academia must be independent of the state, or else freedom of thought and expression would be sacrificed. Leifer, Becker, and others, paid a big price for their courageous acts: they lost and thereafter found it very difficult, if not impossible, to work again in academic psychiatry. For Szasz, here is how he summed it up decades later:

> By 1970, I became a non-person in American psychiatry. The pages of American psychiatric journals were shut to my work. Soon, the very mention of my name became taboo and was omitted from new editions of texts that had previously featured my views. In short, I became the object to that most effective of all criticisms, the silent treatment—or, as the Germans so aptly call it, *Totschweigetaktik* (Szasz, 1997, p. 71).

As history shows, Szasz was not to be denied. He has relentlessly and tirelessly challenged psychiatric coercion.. In so doing, he has become one of the world's leading intellectual voices for liberty and justice. Life is and always has been difficult and risky. Despite loud and voluminous assertions from the kingdom of psychiatry, there are no medical experts who can provide hope and absolution from the challenge of human existence. The false hopes and dangerous practices of psychiatric oppression do far greater harm than good. George Alexander, former dean of the Santa Clara University School of Law, [He was an "assistant dean in Syracuse called Szasz "the greatest freedom fighter of the twentieth century" (Slovenko, 2004, p. 150).

We have all failed thus far to prevent the emergence what Szasz named "the therapeutic state," and we all have our work cut out for us. That Szasz so clearly and powerfully articulated truth, and influenced so many of us, is real and meaningful success. I am one among many who now stand shoulder to shoulder with this man in defense of people as relational individuals, capable of responsibility and good will, entitled to liberty and self-determination. Thomas

Szasz is, to borrow from the Emerson epigraph above, "a declaration of independence walking."

Part II

SZASZIAN PRINCIPLES

John Breeding, PhD

Chapter 1
THE MYTH OF MENTAL ILLNESS

Tom Szasz was the clearest thinker and writer that I have known, and, in general, his influence has been to help me see and think more clearly, especially in regards to my work. It began with *The Myth of Mental Illness* (1961); despite the ongoing massive denial of the undeniable—that the concept of mental illness is a metaphor, and that psychiatry failed 52 years ago, and still fails, to meet the Virchowian standard of disease as a confirmable physical or chemical abnormality in regards to the myriad "mental illnesses" extant today—I have remained crystal clear in seeing the distinction between a metaphor and an objective disease. My ongoing study of Szasz has been vital to withstand the relentless, mind-numbing propaganda in my field. Neurologist Fred Baughman, Jr., a dedicated leader in the struggle to keep this distinction, and its ramifications, clear, has also been a great help and support to me on this. Shortly after Szasz' death, I called Baughman. After we both lamented his passing, Baughman shared with me his frustration about the fact that some of his best allies seemed to be devoting a lot of time and energy to "alternative treatments," mostly nutritional, of things like so-called Attention Deficit Hyperactivity Disorder (ADHD), which Fred has always called a total fraud (Baughman, 2006). It also brings to mind what Szasz said in his book, *Schizophrenia: The Sacred Symbol of Psychiatry* (1976), after pointing out chemist Linus Pauling's (1901-1994) claim that schizophrenia was curable by "megavitamin therapy": "We assume that Pauling accepts his psychiatric colleagues' dictum that what they *call* schizophrenia *is* schizophrenia—a posture that ill becomes a scientist of his stature." (p. 109) Baughman's lament validates the need to do all we can to prevent Szasz's ideas from disappearing in Orwell's "memory hole."

Here is a summary from *Lexicon of Lunacy* on the relevant distinction:

> In short, no psychiatric diagnosis is, or can be, pathology-driven; instead, all such diagnoses are driven by nonmedical (economic, personal, legal, political, and social) factors or incentives. Accordingly, psychiatric diagnoses do not point to pathoanatomic or pathophysiological lesions and do not identify causative agents—but rather refer to human behaviors. Moreover, the psychiatric terms used to refer to such behaviors allude to the plight of the denominated patient, hint at the

dilemmas with which patient and psychiatrist alike try to cope as well as exploit, and mirror the beliefs and values of the society that both inhabit. (Szasz, 1993)

While seeing and understanding that the concept of mental illness is a metaphor, and that psychiatric diagnoses are based strictly on behavior, is vital to clear thinking, it often makes little difference to individuals who are hurting, anxious or depressed, and want medical or financial help or social support—likewise, probably even more so, to those who want someone else to get "help." They frequently don't really care about the scientific validity of the chemical imbalance or bad gene that qualifies them, or the troubling or troubled one they want to get "help" for. On the other hand, I have found the information is deeply appreciated and very helpful to many who have been misled by the ubiquitous propaganda of the industry and the frequent pronouncements of the helping professionals about the biological and/or genetic defects that constitute mental illness. While the industry, represented by groups such as the National Alliance on Mental Illness (NAMI), has campaigns about overcoming the stigma on mental illness—meaning encourage people to accept their disease without shame—I have been honored to support many recovering psychiatric patients who are grateful and empowered to know they really are *not* carrying an organic defect that is a permanent mental illness, and hence meaning permanent treatment, and some degree of disability (Whitaker, 2010). They consistently find liberation from stigma by rejection of the lie of mental illness, not by acceptance of their "disease." In a similar vein, I have had the good fortune of supporting a great many parents, and others, who are immensely relieved and empowered to discover that their children, or other loved ones, are not in fact defective and doomed to a failed and miserable life.

> The point is not that psychiatric diagnoses are meaningless, but that they may be, and often are, swung as semantic blackjacks: cracking the subject's respectability and dignity destroys him just as effectively, and often more so, as cracking his skull. The difference is that the man who wields a blackjack is recognized by everyone as a public menace, but one who wields a psychiatric diagnosis is not. (Szasz, *1966*)

The Myth of Mental Health

So while this piece of information about the distinction between scientific medicine and the pseudoscientific claims of biological psychiatry is crucial, it is the tip of the iceberg in regards to the work of Thomas Szasz. It is also the tip of the spear of the psychiatric industry. Normal necessitates abnormal; if mental illness is a myth, then *mutates mutandis*—as Szasz was wont to say—mental health must also be. And the imperative for mental health professionals is seemingly to restore to health, but actually, given the biopsychiatric belief in the incurability of mental disease, to control the "progression of the illness." The operative word is, of course, control, and the method is the action of "treatment." It is most interesting and illuminating to read Szasz' *Schizophrenia* and learn about the roots of biopsychiatry. In the first chapter, titled "Psychiatry: The Model of the Syphilitic Mind," he points out that at the turn of the 20th century almost a third of asylum inmates were syphilitic. German psychiatrist Emil Kraepelin (1856-1926) invented "demential praecox" in 1898 and Swiss psychiatrist Eugen Bleuler (1857-1939) invented "schizophrenia" in 1911, renaming and expanding the concept. In 1904 German psychiatrist Alois Alzheimer (1864-1915) published the first paper describing the histopathological indicators characteristic of syphilis, and by 1909, German physician Paul Ehrlich (1854-1915) had developed Salvarsan for the treatment of syphilis. Szasz lays out the case that this scientific advance validated and locked in the mindset that continues in psychiatry today—that mental illness is biologically based disease, and that aggressive treatment is necessary for restoration of mental health (even though mental illness is considered incurable!)—and remains impervious to consideration of scientific fact. In any event, the concepts of mental illness and mental health are Siamese twins, inseparable without radical surgery—called "psychiatric treatment"—which will be dangerous, and is often life threatening (Elias, 2007).

In my opinion, one of Szasz's most valuable teachings is that psychiatric diagnoses don't describe anything of real use to individuals or those who want to offer real support. These words from his book, *Schizophrenia*, explain:

> The entire literature on "schizophrenia"—now extending backward in time for nearly seventy [now 100] years, and encompassing hundreds of thousands of "learned" books and essays in all the important languages—is, in my opinion, fatally flawed by a single logical error: namely, all

33

of the contributions to it treat "schizophrenia" if it were the shorthand *description* of a *disease*, when in fact it is the shorthand *prescription* of a disposition; in other words, they use the term *schizophrenia* as if it were a *proposition asserting* something about psychotics, when in fact it is a *justification legitimizing* something that *psychiatrists* do to them. (1976, p. 88).

The point is profound. The core of Szasz's work is about freedom and responsibility—and it is about challenging medicalized oppression (Breeding, 2011). A fundamental piece of oppression theory is that all oppressions entail a claim to virtue that justifies the mistreatment of a specific group of people, simply because they are in that group.

Chapter 2

PSYCHIATRIC OPPRESSION

On Language

Thomas Szasz was a master of language, and of rhetoric; to read his work is to learn and to grow in mental power and wisdom. His prime focus was on psychiatry, but always through the lens of philosophy and ethics for individuals and society. The following short quote provides one powerful guide for me:

> Although linguistic clarification is valuable for individuals who want to think clearly, it is not useful for people whose social institutions rest on the unexamined, literal use of language. (1993, p. 1)

I have humbly discovered, however, that it is one thing to agree with an aphorism, and another to live it. Clarifying language is exceedingly hard work, especially when you are taking on a language into which you have been thoroughly conditioned, and which is put forth in ongoing waves by your profession, the media and now the public at large. I first heard this pithy little statement by humorist Josh Billings (1818-1885) from Szasz, and I remember it because it makes the point so well: "The problem's not that people don't know anything, but that they know so many things that ain't so." And everyone knows about the pains and tragedies of mental illness, and the needs for treatment, and that schizophrenia is genetic, and that depression is caused by a chemical imbalance, and that people in psychiatric hospitals are their for their own good, etc.

In my own self-examination, I have discovered layer upon layer of unexamined language, and my habitual patterns of using words that imply things I don't really believe. I now do better using plain speech instead of psychological jargon, I say "diagnosed as" but don't use diagnoses, and I often recognize questions with underlying assumptions that violate my own beliefs—like "Does my child have ADHD?" Thomas Szasz affected me by his writings for sure, but his greatest influence on me here was indirect, through another close friend and admirer of his, Leonard Roy Frank, a survivor of psychiatric abuse as a young man, and now a leader for decades in the fight for liberation from psychiatric oppression. Frank is known in some literary circles as editor of the *Random House Webster's Quotationary*; relevant to readers of this article, he edited *The History of Shock Treatment* in 1978 and *The Electroshock Quotationary* in 2006. Most especially relevant, Frank worked intensively with Szasz in 2010 and 2011, editing *The Szasz Quotationary*; this is an extraordinary collection, published in October 2011. Frank came by his mastery of language through hard work. For one, he spent years of study recovering from 50 insulin coma shocks and 35 electroshocks, systematically creating loose leaf notebooks, and later computer files, of words that he was relearning. Then over the years he studied Szasz and others, and systematically worked to translate psychiatric jargon into plain speech. I sought Frank out around 1994, when I became active in challenging electroshock, and he became, among other things, my main mentor in examining and simplifying my way of addressing issues in psychology and psychiatry. I learned to speak and write in more or less plain speech, and I still turn to Frank for plain speech checks today. He will have read and commented on my part of this little book before you read it, in addition to contributing the appendix, his selection of Szasz quotations.

Psychiatry as an Agent of Social Control

Psychiatric rhetoric would have us believe that countless people—virtually everyone at some time or other—suffer from mental illness, and that treatment of mental illness is an important, beneficent branch of medicine. Szasz says it's all about power. One of his truly classic works, first published in 1970, is titled, *The Manufacture of Madness: A Comparative Study of the Inquisition and the Mental Health Movement* (1997). This book, perhaps more than any other, helped me understand mental health system oppression. Szasz lays out a fascinating history of the Inquisition, arguing that as we humans shifted from a primarily religious zeitgeist to a scientific worldview, so did the powers that be shift from using religious claims to virtue for their oppressive actions to scientific (medical) claims. Because I was raised Catholic, his analysis was especially meaningful to me. The relevant analogy, derived from the book, is as follows:

> *The Inquisition is to heresy as psychiatry is to mental illness.*

During the Inquisition, the working manual was the *Malleus Maleficarum* (The Hammer of Witches), which affirmed that belief in witches was an essential part of the Catholic faith and, of course, that it was the duty of the inquisitors to act forcefully to save the soul of anyone suspected of being a witch, or otherwise deemed a heretic. As an example of the inquisitors' methods, test by "swimming" was popular in seventeenth century England. The accused witch was restrained and thrown into the water. If she floated, she was guilty; if she sank, she was innocent. That the latter usually resulted in drowning was not a problem since her soul, the inquisitors claimed, went to heaven. Szasz argues that the results of modern diagnostics closely resemble the swimming ordeal. While some witches may have survived dunking, I agree with him that it is the exceedingly rare "madman" who survives psychological testing. My own experience has taught me, for example, that it is the rare child selected out for testing of so-called Attention Deficit Disorder who is not labeled as "mentally ill," and then receives the toxic, dangerous and life-shortening "treatments." Research clearly validates that there is a presumption of "mental illness" by mental health officials, and that it is rare for judges to not go along with a psychiatrist's opinion that an individual needs "treatment." (Scheff, 1984)

The inquisitors presumed guilt; psychiatry presumes mental illness. Just as the claim to virtue for the coercive force of the inquisitors was to save souls, so psychiatrists claim to save minds for the "patient's" own good. That countless Americans are incarcerated in psychiatric institutions every year is testament to the fervor with which psychiatrists impose their so-called "treatments." What makes inquisitors and psychiatrists so dangerous is that in both cases the government authenticates, justifies and in many instances rewards (through insurance payments for example) their actions. These discretionary powers are granted largely due to the fact that Inquisitors and psychiatrists, each in their time, were seen not as punishing persecutors but as their victims' benefactors. Szasz points out that the pious inquisitor would have been outraged at the suggestion that he was the heretic's foe, not his potential savior. In our time, one surefire way to elicit a psychiatrist's rage, is to suggest he is the adversary of his involuntary patient. Whether it is the small heresy of a child failing to fulfill the expectations of school or family, a young person failing to meet the family's expectations of emerging adult independence, or of those we call political dissidents who fail to toe the patriotic line, branding that individual as mentally ill is the way to assert control, and restrict their freedom.

This is a damning analogy; if one takes it to heart, it is necessary to make a profound choice. Do you stand on the side of the inquisitors or with the right of heretics to freedom of thought and expression, and the right to be left alone? Do you use "mental illness" as a justification to treat a person as less than a free moral agent, and curtail their rights to liberty and self-determination? Or do you stand for freedom of belief and action? In all relationships involving people who for whatever reason are perceived as being different, this choice is ever-present, most certainly in everything I do as a psychologist.

The most dramatic deprivation of liberty is total—removal of a citizen from society by incarceration in a state-run, sanctioned or financed facility. Regarding such action, the bottom line for Szasz lies in this one sentence from 1963: "A person should be deprived of liberty only if proved guilty of breaking the law." A large part of his work was devoted to examination of psychiatry and the law.

Part III

PSYCHIATRY AND THE LAW

Chapter 3

PSYCHIATRY AND COERCION

Most counselors avoid overtly dealing with psychiatry and the law, restricting themselves to office appointments; they try to avoid "severe" cases. In reality, even if a counselor insists on refusing anyone who smacks of a potential problem, it is virtually impossible to avoid situations where a client gets into something edgy—a custody problem, a child getting into trouble at school, a client becoming extreme, and especially the problem of suicide, which I will address separately. Given current ethical policies and the current legal practices in society concerning psychiatry, counselors will inevitably face the ethical choices that Szasz laid out.

One simple yet important example lies in the question of privacy. Privacy concerns are central in psychology and psychiatry, and no less so for Szasz. He believed and practiced an absolute standard of privacy in the contract between himself and his clients. In the modern world of "mental health services," privacy has been severely, often totally, compromised. It is routine practice to report to insurance companies, to child protective services, to courts and lawyers, to government agencies, to family members, to just about anyone. One common denominator has to do with who is paying the "provider." Szasz was aghast at such arrangements, and I would urge anyone who is uncertain or has not thought deeply about this slippery slope to spend some time with Szasz's writings. Later in this paper I will discuss more on his views on counseling; regarding psychiatry and the law, it is sufficient to point out that when a "mental health professional" acts as an agent of the state in legal proceedings "in the best interests of"—really against—an individual defendant ("patient"), privacy is not even in the game.

Psychiatry and Children

It is actually quite common for counselors to deal with the law. One example is when there is any kind of actual or potential involvement of state protective services, for children in situations where there is any suspicion of abuse or neglect. Given that judgments in these instances are quite subjective, especially in cases of neglect, which constitute the majority of child protective service cases, this comes up frequently for those who work with children and families. The straight up ethics policy is a demand to report in any suspected case; once one takes a close look at the limits and problems with actual child protective service agency practices, however, it is not so simple (Baughman and Breeding, 2003). Adult protective service agency concerns can come into play as well.

One situation I frequently encounter involves parents reaching out or taking action in response to their "problem child." My entry into private counseling in the 1980's just happened to correlate with the pharmaceutical industry's discovery of children as a largely untapped market for psychiatric drugs, the invention of ADD in 1980 and ADHD in 1987 by the American Psychiatric Association and the subsequent discovery and diagnosis of millions of school-age children needing treatment with stimulant drugs (Breeding, 2007). My need to respond to this phenomenon was a significant catalyst for my political activism, and it has been my pleasure to disrupt this action on many an occasion and to offer a decent alternative to many adults in parenting their challenging children. One specific decision as a counselor is whether you will work with families who choose to give psychiatric drugs to their children. I don't, unless it is to support them in thinking and deciding on actions to wean their children and go down a different road.

A most significant place that the law comes in regarding psychiatric labeling and drugging of children is in the educational system through the Individuals with Disabilities Education Act (IDEA), which in 1991 added ADHD as a qualifying disability for special education monies and services. Coercion does come into play here as many parents are pressured to diagnose and drug their children, and many struggle with a felt need to get a diagnosis in order to qualify a child for special education resources and accommodations. I have often consulted with parents in this situation, and I consider it my moral duty to engage in serious conversation. This selection of children is a very slippery slope, an example of the "therapeutic state" that Szasz challenges (Szasz, 1984), one that has resulted in huge numbers of people on welfare for psychiatric disability in the United States (Whitaker, 2010). One choice for a psychologist is to make disability evaluations and help people qualify; another is to choose not to participate in that kind of activity and to seriously consider the ramifications, especially from the Szaszian point of view about autonomy and responsibility.

I was so troubled by the drugging of children in the schools, and by the coercion, that I became very involved in lobbying for two laws that were passed in Texas in 2003; one made it illegal for teachers and other school personnel to suggest a diagnosis or recommend a drug for a child; the other made it illegal for Child Protective Services (CPS) to accuse a parent of medical neglect for refusing to administer a psychotropic drug to their child (Breeding, 2003). Related to the involvement of CPS, I have also worked with a number of divorced parents who wanted help with challenging a co-parent, often in a regrettably hostile situation, who was already administering psychiatric drugs to their child or wanting to. I don't often choose to get involved in custody battles, but in these cases, I will do what I can to support the parent who wants to protect their child from the drugs.

While Szasz did not write a lot about children and families, here is an excerpt from a short speech he gave a few years back that summarizes his position:

> Labeling a child is stigmatization, not diagnosis. Giving a child a psychiatric drugs is poisoning, not treatment. I have long maintained that the child psychiatrist is one of the most dangerous enemies not only of children, but of adults, of all of us who care to the most precious and most vulnerable things in life. And those two things are children and liberty. (Szasz, 2008)

Psychiatry's Twin Pillars of Power: Involuntary Commitment and The Insanity Defense

Another common experience I have had is when a parent has the urge to, or actually does call in the state—the police, usually, sometimes mental health deputies—on an older child who is "acting out," or judged as being in distress. In the former, it is often possible to help avoid such an action with a little encouragement, information and support. The latter very often involves supporting the parent to process regret and disillusionment at the results of thinking that the state can do a better job for their family then they can. There is often a rude awakening to the fact that, once the state is involved, choice is gone or at least greatly limited, and one is at the mercy of the psychiatrists in charge. I have also seen this in situations where an adult voluntarily enters a psychiatric facility, only to experience the truth that once inside, you can leave only when a psychiatrist says you can, not when you want to. There can be no truly voluntary psychiatry as long as involuntary commitment remains an option for the family or psychiatrist. I also often counsel adults who want to work on recovering from the effects of trauma suffered at the hands of the mental health system, and I do provide non-medical support for some who have decided to wean themselves off psychiatric drugs. Much of the latter involves working through fear, shame, hopelessness, and the false belief

43

that they will necessarily deteriorate if they discontinue taking these drugs; these are residual effects of psychiatric labeling and treatment (Breeding, 1998).

Nevertheless, I think most psychologists think of themselves as not being involved with psychiatry and the law, considering that the domain of the forensic psychology specialty, where "experts" do evaluations and testify on issues of insanity and competency. Szasz wrote extensively on these dynamics (1965, 1970, 1987) as they speak to the heart of his abhorrence at the egregious violations of liberty perpetrated by this system. Since I took a stand in alignment with him on this issue, agreeing with the aphoristic title of historian Howard Zinn's autobiography *You Can't Be Neutral on a Moving Train,* I have been involved in many cases of technically legal psychiatric coercion. Oftentimes, it has been as simple as testifying at a state hospital commitment hearing. If you attend a few of these hearings, and think about what you are observing, two things quickly become obvious. First, the rituals of court, with judge, prosecutor and defense attorney, sure do look like criminal proceedings. Szasz' quip that to verify disease, regular doctors use pathologists, but psychiatrists use lawyers is tragically apt.

Psychiatrists don't use pathologists to verify mental illness because they can't. As Szasz wisely put it,

> Psychiatrists insist that schizophrenia and manic-depressive psychosis are brain diseases. Textbooks of pathology describe and discuss all known bodily diseases, including brain diseases. Accordingly, one way to verify whether schizophrenia and manic-depressive psychosis are brain diseases is to see what the authors of textbooks of pathology say about them. Well, the fact is that they do not say anything about these alleged diseases: they do not mention them, as they simply do not recognize mental illnesses as bodily diseases. (1987, p. 71)

Second, you would notice the fact that the deal is rigged; it is rare for the psychiatrist's opinion not to win out. I have been involved with several cases where my showing up and testifying, especially after consulting with the defense attorney and encouraging a real defense (as opposed to the general practice of mostly collaborating with the prosecutor "for the patient's own good"), actually resulted in a judge's decision to release the defendant. I will briefly discuss three specific cases in chapters 4, 5 and 6.

If one works with people accused of being seriously mentally ill—as I sometimes do—things often get very thorny, as issues of competency and "dangerousness to self and others" come into play. It is impossible to determine the number of Americans who are forcibly incarcerated in psychiatric institutions for long or short periods of time every year, but they are surprisingly large. Based on extrapolation from a California sampling in the latter 1980's a conservative estimate is 1.5 million, a testament to the fervor of such "treatment." (Citizens Commission on Human Rights, 1994) The flip side of such widespread "involuntary commitment" is the insanity defense. The following from Szasz summarizes the dynamics of psychiatry's twin pillars of power:

> Why do we talk about the rights of mental patients? Who threatens or abridges them? The answer is painfully obvious: relatives, physicians, psychiatrists, judges, legislators — all those responsible for the complex web of images, justifications, and policies that result in institutional psychiatry and its involuntary patients. Commitment, involuntary mental hospitalization, is, of course, the paradigm of psychiatric power. In my opinion, it is also a paradigm of the perversion of power: for if the "patient" is not a criminal, then he or she has a right to liberty; and if the patient is a criminal, then he or she ought to be restrained and punished by the criminal law, like anyone else....

> Involuntary mental hospitalization and the insanity defense should be seen for what they are: symmetrical symbols of psychiatric power. In the one case, the psychiatrist "accuses" the innocent; in the other, he "excuses" the guilty. Civil commitment and the insanity defense both create and confirm the impression of psychiatric expertise, where none exists. Civil commitment and the insanity defense also foster the impression that they provide a socially beneficial solution for troubling problems of human existence, when, actually both aggravate these problems. In short, both are inimical to, and indeed incompatible with, the principles of a free society. (1982)

I think a family member initiates the most common path to psychiatric incarceration, but anyone can call in the police and/or mental health deputies, express a concern, report a disturbance, and start the process. The fact that it is, in some ways in some places, a bit more difficult to get someone committed today than in times past—and a little easier to challenge someone's commitment if help is mobilized—is owing to a significant degree to the ongoing, relentless ruckus Szasz has made in arguing for liberty and due process rights for citizens, even those accused of being mentally ill. Nevertheless, the commitment mill runs full-time, and it goes on mostly unchecked. It is a way to deal with troubled or troubling conduct that falls short of criminality, and it is generally a two-step process involving incarceration and drugging. While court proceedings for these two events are officially separate, they tend to be handled concurrently, or in rapid succession; since psychiatry today means biopsychiatry, mental illness means psychiatric drugs as treatment. Both incarceration and drugging are forced assaultive actions, but each is called medical treatment—hence, the apt title of Szasz's book on the history of psychiatry, *Coercion as Cure* (2007).

Chapter 4

THE CASE OF SOHRAB HASSAN

The experience I had in the case of Sohrab Hassan, described in some detail in an earlier publication (Breeding, 2006), illustrates many relevant points. First, his brothers were concerned about his behavior and convinced him to get psychiatric help, which he did in September 2004. After being under a local psychiatrist's care for several months, Hassan discontinued the drug treatment. His brothers initiated police visits, which resulted in the police leaving after judging him to be rational and peaceful. But then the brothers, together with the psychiatrist, escalated their efforts to control him by convincing the sheriff's department to present Mr. Hassan with an order of protective custody, which means temporary incarceration in a psychiatric facility. So there was some resistance by the police to the brothers' desires, but soon enough Hassan was locked up against his will, though no crimes have been mentioned or charged. The next step would be a commitment hearing, but along the way, Hassan had a highly unusual experience. While he was at the psychiatric institution, he talked with and made friends with one of his fellow "patients"—a woman who was there voluntarily. The woman was there less than 24 hours as she very quickly decided that she had made a bad decision to go to this place for help, and was allowed to leave. This was fortunate for her and, as it turns out, for Hassan. For the woman was a criminal defense attorney, and when he then called her and asked for her help, she took his case. Ironically, the woman's assigned psychiatrist was the same man who had "treated" Hassan voluntarily as an outpatient, and was now determined to "treat" him against his will while he was incarcerated. The lawyer called me, and we went to court.

Sohrab Hassan had a kind of help that is very rarely available in these kinds of cases; he had a real criminal defense attorney who had the ironic advantage of no experience with mental health law and proceedings. This is an advantage because she understood that legal proceedings in this country are antagonistic, and acted accordingly—she had absolutely no illusions that the psychiatrist was acting as a doctor to help his patient; rather, he was an adversary attempting to incarcerate this man and subject hi to unwanted "treatment." It was good to watch this as a real fight, though discouraging that we lost the hearing and Hassan was committed (jailed) for up to 90 days because he was deemed so severely mentally ill that he was dangerous to himself and others.

A second hearing on forced drugging ("court-ordered medication") was delayed for several days, during which period the "patient" was allowed to refuse medication. This hearing was intense, and the amazing thing is that we won. I think I did my part as I have learned with experience how to deal effectively with prosecutors. One key is refusing, while testifying as an expert witness, to answer questions on the prosecutor's terms. She would set up yes-or-no questions, such as "Do you believe in mental illness?" or "Would you ever think medication was a good idea if Mr. Hassan was seriously mentally ill?" While I do have a direct answer, in this context, either yes or no is damning. The one supports her case, the other paints me as a fringe radical in the eyes of the court—to effectively answer the question in this context requires laying out a discussion of what these terms mean. On the one hand, I would bring the focus back to Hassan, and on the other, I would expand on the concept of mental illness, and the issue of safety and efficacy of various kinds of help.

A memorable experience was when the prosecutor asked me point blank whether I would rather see Mr. Hassan butt-raped in prison than receive the psychiatric treatment he needed for his mental illness. This theme runs very deep in the mental health courts. A major claim to virtue is that the state taking beneficent psychiatric care of these mentally ill people is so much kinder and gentler than harsh judicial trial, sentencing and doing time in prison. In any event, the judge ruled that Sohrab Hassan was competent to refuse medication and disallowed the petition. She did go on an extended lecture to the defendant, which had the feel of a rant, about her certainty that even though she had to concede he had the legal right to refuse medication, that this was a bad decision. She particularly emphasized that it would look so much better for his criminal cases—pending misdemeanor charges of trespass and DWI—if he were to show the judge and prosecutor that he was taking medication for his mental illness. This judge could use a Szasz tutorial herself, perhaps starting with this quotation:

> We should not forget the value inherent in the right to be tried — in *public* and by one's own *peers,* and also the values inherent in the right to go to jail — instead of being subjected to unwanted psychiatric "treatments." In a jail, a person is "let alone"; in a mental hospital he may not be. A prisoner will be released after he completes his sentence, and possibly before. A mental patient may be required to

undergo a change in his "inner personality" — a change that may be induced by measures far more intrusive than anything permitted in a jail — before the psychiatric authorities let him go. And they may never let him go. Commitment, unlike a sentence, is for an indefinite period.

How different the world might be today if only a handful of people had been sent for psychiatric "treatments," instead of being tried and sent to jail! Gandhi, Nehru, Sukarno, Castro, Hitler — and of course many others, for example the "freedom riders" in the South — have been sentenced to terms in prison. Surely, the social *status quo* could have been better preserved by finding each of these men mentally ill and subjecting them to enough electric shock treatments to quell their aspirations. If this is not the kind of tyranny against which the Constitution was intended to protect us, what is? (Szasz, 1963)

It is powerfully revealing that despite being adjudicated as seriously and dangerously mentally ill and "committed" for 90 days in the first hearing, Sohrab Hassan was discharged from Seton Shoal Creek Hospital a few days later, immediately upon return from the second hearing. It appears that psychiatry today has little to offer beyond drugs and the backup of electroshock. I also think that these places do not like so much attention.

John Breeding, PhD

Chapter 5

THE CASE OF RODNEY YODER

Psychiatrists and the courts serve a political function of defining power and control in society. However, most times they are responding to the daily dramas of family struggles and conflicts, as compared to dealing with overtly political power politics. These cases do happen, however, even within my own limited experience. One is the case of Rodney Yoder. Alaska attorney James Gottstein's (2001) legal memo is a good summary of Yoder's case up to that time. I just want to make a few brief points here. In December 2002, I testified at Yoder's commitment hearing in Illinois. The situation, according to court records, was that the public was protected from a very dangerous, psychotic man via the mechanisms of law and psychiatry; he had been held under a series of involuntary commitment orders since July of 1991, over a decade, after completing a short prison stay on an assault charge. His psychiatric hospitalization was considered necessary for the safety of the public, and for Yoder's own good. This was reaffirmed in the 2002 trial, despite a strong effort by attorney Randy Kretchmar, and the testimony of Fred Baughman and myself among others.

The biggest challenge to the official story consists of the presence of Rodney Yoder. Yoder consistently and persistently refused to acknowledge his "illness" or cooperate with the authorities in any way. He called his hospitalization imprisonment, the doctors his captors and the treatment they forced on him torture. He demonstrated his mental competence by arguing and winning various legal appeals during incarceration. He organized the mobilization of a significant movement of activists on the outside, including recruitment of a lawyer and "experts" like Baughman and myself. All this was accomplished mostly with letters scrawled in pencil from his prison cell. During the December trial, I was privileged to observe the demonstration of Yoder's intellectual competence in the testimony he gave. Throughout the stressful situation, Yoder kept his cool and delivered the best treatise on the theory and practice of psychiatric oppression I'd ever heard from anyone other than Thomas Szasz.

There is a clear presumption of guilt when it comes to declarations of mental illness by a psychiatrist, and prosecutors and judges are generally very strong about the inability of persons deemed mentally ill to determine their own best interests. No matter how clear and rational a person may seem, they are disregarded. If the person is a bit emotional or "inappropriate," it becomes even easier to condescendingly disregard; if the person accuses his helpers of torture and torment, and calls his "hospital" a psychoprison as Yoder did, he is most definitely severely mentally ill. And if on top of that, he coolly and intelligently lays out a Szaszian analysis before a kangaroo court, he is even crazier and more dangerous.

An important truth about any trial situation is that experts are compromised because both sides will buy an expert who states their opinion. As a result, each side cancels out the other. On this particular battle of challenging the validity of biopsychiatry, however, just as in the courts in general, it gets even worse in that so often the challengers have to work on a volunteer basis since defendants are usually poor and therefore unable to hire attorneys and expert witnesses to take their side. The state or the insurance or drug companies, on the other hand, have the financial resources to hire experts, often the best that money can buy. For example, the state spent at least $100,000 on the December involuntary commitment trial for Rodney Yoder, and the defense consisted of a volunteer lawyer and experts. In the end, the result tends to be the same since the judges are agents of the state whose job is to defend customary and usual practice. Anyone who could see and hear Yoder during that trial, and who still declares him dangerously mentally ill, simply cannot and/or will not see reality for what it is. The reality those jurors (all inhabitants of a town almost totally dependent on the prison industry) see is mightily distorted.

Chapter 6

THE CASE OF CAROLYN BARNES

I want to discuss in more detail one last case in which I was involved, regarding what seems to be overt use of legal psychiatric coercion for political purposes as it clearly exposes the tragic farce. Before proceeding, however, it is important to add a third, related column to Szasz' twin pillars of involuntary commitment and the insanity defense—what might be considered a mutant hybrid of the two. The hybrid has to do with judgments of competency to stand trial, and the resultant "treatment" is called "competency restoration." Of late in Texas, we are seeing this with a number of our citizens as they are declared incompetent to stand trial, and shuttled off to state psychiatric facilities for so-called competency restoration. In common with involuntary commitment, citizens are incarcerated without a trial, without any conviction of law-breaking. In common with the insanity defense, they are presumed incompetent and incapable of understanding, and locked up indefinitely without trial. The recent surge in Texas notwithstanding, this is actually not a new dynamic; Szasz addressed it in detail in his 1965 book, *Psychiatric Justice*, in which he describes the state's use of "psychiatric hospitalization because of unfitness to stand trial" by demonstrating "how the modern state may use psychiatry as a weapon against the individual citizen." (p. 11). One gem of this book is the record of trial transcripts in which Szasz testified; these New York cases from 50 years past sound just like the case of Carolyn Barnes that I will introduce here. (Breeding, 2012)

A very brief background is that Carolyn Barnes has been a liberty-loving activist attorney in Williamson County for many years. In May of 2010, Barnes was arrested and charged with assault for allegedly firing a gun at a census worker. The case is full of holes, not the least of which is that an eyewitness has her elsewhere than on the property where the alleged incident took place. Some of Barnes' many friends and supporters have created a blog that lays out enough of her case to give the interested reader more detail (Free Carolyn Barnes, 2012).

The bigger issue, though, is that the guilt or innocence of Carolyn Barnes is irrelevant. From the very beginning, June of 2010, she has been denied her right to an examining trial and speedy jury trial, and eventually denied her right to an attorney of her choosing or to represent herself. The legal issues of the case are complex, but the situation really broke down at a scheduled jury trial on February   28, 2011, when Barnes requested a continuance in order to secure the exculpatory evidence the State was refusing to produce, and the visiting judge said that he would grant the continuance for four months only if she accepted a court-appointed attorney.   The visiting judge then summarily revoked her bond without warning, and put her back in jail with no bond, where she was kept in solitary confinement for more than three months, until being summarily declared incompetent to stand trial and sent to the maximum security unit at the North Texas State Hospital for the criminally insane. There she was repeatedly beat up by another inmate, and after the better part of a year there, was transferred to Kerrville State Hospital, where she seemed safe from brutalization, but continued to be locked up without recourse to justice.

Finally, after 15 months in state psychiatric prisons, Barnes was told she would have a "competency hearing." Less than two weeks prior to Szasz's death, on August 28, 2012, I sat in a Williamson County courthouse for Barnes' hearing, and witnessed one of the greatest travesties of justice and affronts to liberty I have ever seen. First of all, it was supposed to be a jury trial, and her right to that had already been abolished by an agreement between the prosecutor, judge and Barnes' court-appointed "defense" attorney. Her right to the attorney of her choice, or to represent herself, was of course also disregarded as the judge had ordered the same attorney originally chosen for her prior to the February 2011 aborted trial. This was the same man who had betrayed Barnes by advocating for the declaration of incompetence because she rejected his insistence that she plea-bargain. So in Barnes' case, defense and prosecution were working together, which is unusual because prosecutors commonly order evaluation of competence by a state-sponsored psychiatrist. While this makes it even more obvious that psychiatrists often serve as agents of the state, the result is the same—the evaluating psychiatrist is presented as the patient's doctor when in fact he or she is working for the state prosecution in a legal adversarial position. Barnes' case is one definitive instance where the obfuscation of this distinction bears tragic fruit.

The judge ignored Ms. Barnes' very calm and considered pleas and objections, treating her mostly as a non-entity—another clear demonstration that labeling someone as mentally ill is the most effective way to create a non-citizen with limited rights of autonomy and self-determination, hardly any legal rights, and no worthiness of respect for his or her own ideas and wishes. Barnes' Kerrville psychiatrist, Janet True, refused to comment on her competence, but said she did need continued treatment as she was now suffering from a major depressive disorder. This psychiatrist also testified that Barnes was not a danger to anyone. The prosecutors never presented any testimony that she was incompetent to stand trial, which was the sole purpose of the hearing.

Barnes did manage to get me on the stand and I explained that my continued interaction with Barnes for the last two years was consistent with the evaluation I wrote in June 2010—which the court had never allowed into testimony. I initially evaluated Barnes in person. During her incarceration, I kept in regular touch with her by phone and through correspondence. At the hearing, I testified that Barnes was very intelligent, clear, articulate, with deep understanding of her own case and of the law in general; in short, she was, and is exceedingly competent.

What's going on? Barnes, and many of her activist friends and former clients, explain that she has been a thorn in the side of the Williamson County powers for some time. They are certain that this is a way to put her out of commission. Barnes is convinced that her incarceration began as a vendetta by district attorney John Bradley. As with Rodney Yoder, I tend to believe Barnes, but my beliefs in that regard are irrelevant. Her case is an example of psychiatric coercion, of control exerted by accusations of "madness" in order to evade justice. Fundamental rights to a fair and speedy trial, to the lawyer of your choice, and countless other constitutional guarantees have been repeatedly and systematically trampled during her incarceration for over 20 months. The involved psychiatrist and the jurists have betrayed their functions, and the human rights of Barnes, all in the name of protection, help and "therapy."

Regardless of how her legal problems started, the curtailment of Barnes' rights to due process and the resultant indefinite detention are a massive violation. They rendered her into nonpersonhood. It is painful to witness this kind of tragedy, and such pain is one reason why more people do not see past the claims to virtue of psychiatric oppression. In any event, once that road to psychiatric perdition is open, emerging from the locked gates is excruciatingly difficult. For one thing, when a citizen fights back, the oppressors often escalate their repressiveness because backing down means losing face and risking legal action against them and all manner of potential liability. There was an Austin American Statesman newspaper reporter present at the August hearing. While his report skirted the ethical issues, at least it describes a terrible insult to injury that we are seeing more. In his article, Eric Dexheimer (10/20/12) reported on the fact that the state is not only forcibly "treating" Barnes against her will, but also billing her for the services; here is how Dexheimer begins his article:

> Carolyn Barnes received her latest hospital bill on Oct. 3. "Dear Ms. Barnes," it said. "You owe the Kerrville State Hospital $97,728 as reimbursement for the support, maintenance and treatment it provided to you for dates of service March 20, 2012 through September 30, 2012." If the bill was not paid or successfully challenged, the letter continued, the hospital would file a lien against Barnes' property.

On Wednesday, January 9, 2013, Carolyn Barnes was put into handcuffs and transferred from Kerrville State hospital to the Williamson County jail. The state hospital staff and a state contract psychologist both decided she is now competent to stand trial. Two days later, the Williamson County court held another competency hearing and Judge Shaver declared her competent. Despite strong assurances and evidence that she was neither dangerous or a flight risk, and that she was broke after two years in custody, he set bail at $30,000 and required that Barnes wear an ankle monitor. (Dexheimer, 2013) Even though her ordeal continued, there was cause for muted celebration because she made bail the next day with contributions from friends and supporters. The criminal charges were eventually adjudicated that spring.

It is worth briefly considering why Barnes was declared competent in January, but not in August. As I testified again in the January hearing, my judgment was that she has always been competent. General factors that often make a difference, and were present in Barnes' case, were recent media attention to her travails, and recent visits to Kerrville by allies, including two men from the Citizens Commission on Human Rights who spoke with authorities there concerning possible problems with the handling of her case. Having allies, and both newspaper and television reporters at the hearings also helped a great deal. She got a new attorney in October, Todd Dudley, who proved to be an effective advocate who fought hard on her behalf. The pressure of the various appeals Barnes had filed was another big factor as Williamson County liability may have been greater with continued incarceration and the avoidance of due process. The replacement of the district attorney,

John Bradley, who started the actions against Barnes, is another factor.

In June 2013, Barnes finally had a trial on her original charges of shooting at a census worker. She was convicted and sentenced to three years in prison. I will not comment here on that trial, but however fair or unfair it should have happened in 2010.

Another obstacle to liberation from psychiatric oppression is that once tagged as "mad" (be it mentally ill or incompetent), one's actions and words are systematically ignored and used against you whenever possible. Once a "mental patient," once locked up in a psychiatric facility, no matter the reason or validity, one is ex post facto mentally sick. Further, those tainted by association with a mentally ill person are also discredited. As Szasz put it, "suspicions of the law about mental competence are extended to all those the accused himself considers his agents or friends" (1965, p. 23); this is one more small price to pay for associating and embracing the ideas and practices of Thomas Szasz.

Whatever one's opinion about the personalities or characters of Rodney Yoder and Carolyn Barnes, they are persons of courage and principle—both refused to plea bargain, both refused to play the game of passive acquiescence that is often advised to gain release from psychiatric prisons, both successfully resisted the pressure to force drugs on them, both took the legal and PR fight to their opponents as best they could with a severely stacked deck against them. I have observed that people like Barnes and Yoder often pay a high price for their principled actions, just as a slave who refused to shine on his masters (Szasz, 2002), or in fact any citizen who chooses an act of civil disobedience in regards to any social injustice.

John Breeding, PhD

Chapter 7

ON CRITICISM OF THOMAS SZASZ

Before delving into "practicing Szasz" as a counselor per se, I want to comment on criticism of Szasz by his colleagues. Such criticism is vast (Schaler, 2004), and reflects the degree of threat that psychiatrists believe his ideas pose to their profession. While there are many specific criticisms I think they tend to boil down to two main ones—that Szasz lacks compassion for the "mentally ill," and that he is an old-school dinosaur who denies or fails to understand the modern consensus opinion on the nature of mind and body. His defense of an outdated Cartesian split of mind and body negates, in their view, the advances psychiatry has made in diagnosing and treating the mentally ill.

As a practicing psychologist who mostly agrees with Szasz, I face many of the same criticisms. When I am on the front lines at the legislature challenging mental health screening and "suicide prevention" because I see it mostly as a marketing tool for Big Pharma, and as a dangerous threat to our young people, I am in direct opposition to most of my profession, which accepts the rhetoric that such screening is an effort to find and meet the needs of mentally ill children. I am accused of being uncompassionate. The same goes with challenging psychiatry and the law, as discussed above—witness my interaction with the prosecutor about rape in the case of Sohrab Hassan. When I point out the important distinction between diagnosing illness by confirmation of a physical or chemical abnormality and diagnosing "illness" by judging behavior, I am also accused of denying the above said teachings about the unity of mind and body. Practicing Szasz requires the development of psychological and linguistic muscle, and it helps to have a few excellent allies. Reading Szasz, and befriending some of the folks in the circle of Szasz-oriented allies, is a fundamental aid in such development.

The first criticism—that Szasz lacks compassion—is made of all libertarians, and reflects a basic argument heard again and again in political discussions; the polarity is presented as "bleeding heart liberals" and "self-centered conservatives." But as with most polarities, when explored with a little depth it is not nearly so clear. Szasz was a self-declared libertarian, but he also declared himself a classical liberal; this latter means he valued democracy and freedom and liberty of the individual to make choices and live accordingly. The state's role would be to put controls only where resulting actions directly interfere with the constitutional rights of others.

Szasz's great sin was his conviction that rights of liberty should apply to all, not just those who escaped the judgment of psychiatry that they were mentally ill. The title of his book, *Cruel Compassion* (1994), aptly summarizes his conviction that coercion is cruel, no matter the rhetoric. My own experience is that regrettably few people have read Szasz, and so most criticism has no real validity. I can say that reading Szasz has left me with a feeling that he is compassionate. I found it most interesting to discover his summation of *The Myth of Psychotherapy* (1978) wherein he referred to psychotherapy as "the secular cure of souls," (p. 208) and adapted the words of Aeschylus referring to the use of healing words to recommend the term *iatrologic* to replace psychotherapy for the profession of counseling.

Szasz was tough, but he was also kind. I agree with him that state coercion is a cruel assault on liberty, and to call it otherwise is an Orwellian justification of oppression. Regarding opinions on Szasz, I defer to my friend Leonard Frank knew Szasz well, and last week when remembering him, simply said how good-hearted a man he was. The following quote is just one glimpse into the caring heart of Szasz:

> If the Other's affliction lies in his soul rather than his body, then our urge to help him cannot be satisfied without our feeling empathy for him, without our establishing a bond of intimacy with him. (1993)

As to the second criticism that Szasz clung to an old Cartesian paradigm, I never had a chance to ask Szasz about it, but I would certainly never call him naive. Regardless, his main focus was always in challenging oppression, and the rhetoric that justifies it. As a true libertarian, Szasz stood firmly and consistently on the principle of allowing people to choose foolish and dangerous ways, including things like licit and illicit drugs and electroshock, as long as it was a free choice. But to lie and mislead people about illness, and to use such lies to justify the practice of a false medicine is both fraudulent and harmful. To stand by and refuse to say otherwise is cruel and unethical. Moral and linguistic clarification requires a distinction between the nature of mind and body. And when a physical or chemical abnormality is demonstrably present, such is not "mental illness," but physical, even when the symptoms are reflected in thought and behavior. It really is that simple.

In my view it is actually a cruel irony that those who argue that insistence on an "outdated, anachronistic mind-body dualism"— such as Szasz, Baughman and myself propose—is both ignorant and harmful also tend to undermine the spiritual and psychological realities of human existence. Szasz intensely challenged coercion and defended liberty; he also intensely challenged and defended the moral, relational and psychological spheres of human life. His ideas help me stay strong in my conviction that psychological distress and problems in living are not best understood as due to underlying biological or genetic defects, but have their roots in the often harsh realities of existence on the one hand, and in the nature of the human psyche and its vulnerabilities on the other. Deferral to an unproven biopsychiatric explanation and response is not only used to weirdly justify coercion, but also tends to utterly undermine the need and value of counseling. Furthermore, it undermines the autonomy and responsibility of the individual, the value of which was always central to Szasz, and to ethical respectful counseling. As in all areas, to explore Szasz's teachings on counseling, one has to explore (read) his work, but I will say a little more about it in the next section.

Part IV

ON COUNSELING

Chapter 8

PRACTICING SZASZ AS A COUNSELOR

Privacy and Autonomy

I mentioned above the absolute value of privacy in Szasz' life and ideas, most especially in regards to counseling. In researching this book, I read Szasz's 1965 book, *The Ethics of Psychoanalysis: The Theory and Method of Autonomous Psychotherapy*, in which he used the term autonomous psychotherapy, and laid out the principles of such an approach. Szasz wrote that, "autonomy is the only positive freedom whose realization does not injure others" (p. 22), further asserting the requirement of a voluntary, private contract for such a relationship. I was fascinated to discover that Szasz viewed psychoanalysis as a big step forward in support of individual freedom. He argued that "Freud devised a method of psychotherapy to extend the patient's autonomy and named it 'psychoanalysis'," even while he railed against that same name applying to procedures that at the time of his writing, and obviously still today, curtail autonomy. I have been "practicing Szasz" for many years, but reading *The Ethics of Psychoanalysis* has already helped me to stress the importance of clients' taking responsibility for their actions as a way to enhance their autonomy. Based on my reading of Szasz, I know my own approach to counseling is different from his in some ways, as of course it must be. As an example, although a review of his writing on psychoanalysis affirms that Szasz saw the value of catharsis, in general he did not write much about emotion. In contrast, I often do emphasize emotional discharge in my work; I also often focus on trauma and sometimes do transpersonal work.

In an interview with *Reason* editor Jacob Sullum, Szasz had this to say in a response to a query about his approach to therapy:

> To me the whole idea of calling it "therapy" is crippling. So there was a kind of understanding between the other person and me that we were having a conversation about what he could do with his life. That obviously involves adopting different tenets of sorts—different ways of relating to his wife, his children, his job. The premise was that the only person who could change the person was the person himself. My role was as a catalyst. You are making suggestions and exploring alternatives—helping the

> person change himself. The idea that the person remains entirely in charge of himself is a fundamental premise. (Sullum, 2000)

I, too, dislike the term therapy and for similar reasons, so I use the word counseling instead. In any event, one fundamental point that can hardly be overstated in considering counseling is the ongoing, pervasive impact of the structure of the modern "mental health system," in particular the hierarchy of a medical model that positions psychiatrists as the alpha dogs. In *The Myth of Psychotherapy* (1978), chapter 5 begins with this sentence: "The psychotherapist's identity rests on that of the psychiatrist." (p. 67) Of course, the psychiatrist's identity rests on the presumed existence of mental illnesses as medical entities, which he is said to treat.

On Power

In the 2000 interview quoted above, Sullum asked whether psychiatrists have more or less power than they used to have. Szasz's response should give pause to thoughtful counselors, "mental health professionals":

> I think they have much, much more power, but it has become increasingly covert and subtle. If you focus on psychiatrists per se, then perhaps they have a little less power, but the power has been diffused among "mental health professionals": school psychologists, grief counselors, drug treatment specialists, and so on. It pervades society. Sixty years ago, when I went to medical school, this kind of activity was limited entirely to psychiatrists.

> So traditional psychiatrists may have less power. They certainly don't have the feudal slave estates of the old state hospitals, where the patients were washing their cars. That's gone. On the other hand, there is a Tocquevillean kind of oppression—a softer kind of totalitarianism.

Iatrogenic Trauma

There are a great many ways in which counselors are affected by the structure of our mental health system, but much of it can be described this way. In counselor training, one learns about theories of behavior and distress, and theories of counseling. The nuts and bolts of counseling tend to be about personal anguish and trauma, and relationships and such—the effects of how we have been hurt. What most powerfully shook me up when I started professional counseling about 30 years ago was the presence of a whole other level of hurt; I was witnessing in my clients a parade of people who had been hurt by the very people they had reached out to, or been sent to, for help—that is, my fellow mental health professionals. Sometimes it was the stuff that is agreed upon as unethical by the vast majority, and certainly by the official ethics committees of the professional associations—things like sexual relationships between a counselor and client. More often, though, it was the effect of "customary and usual practice," such as the ubiquitous use of psychotropic drugs, and the less frequent but all too common electroshock. There was, of course, the bane of Szasz' life work, coercion and its destructive effects. It is amazing how many people can and do think they are still functioning as counselors, as opposed to jailers, when they work with people who have been forced to see them. Most pervasive are two things that many people do not even see, and that reading Szasz is a magnificent aid in gaining the eyes to see. These are the debilitating effects on everyone involved—client, counselor, friends and family—of believing in the myth of mental illness and the inherent defects entailed, and the undermining of autonomy and responsibility. I am absolutely aligned with Szasz in this aspect of his views on counseling:

> The goal is to assume more responsibility and therefore gain more liberty and more control over one's own life. The issues or questions for the patient become to what extent is he willing to recognize his evasions of responsibility, often expressed as "symptoms." (Wyatt, 2000)

Talking and Listening

To me, this short quote is consistent with my reading of Szasz, in which I see a consistent deliberate eschewal of power and control as a counselor, and a genuine humility. I like Barry Duncan and Scott Miller's research on counseling effectiveness. In their book,

The Heroic Client (2000), they show that the single biggest factor in determining counseling outcomes is "extratherapeutic," meaning that it has nothing to do with the counseling per se, but is a result of things the client does outside of counseling. I think Szasz knew this, and that even if it were not true, he still would have insisted that such an attitude was the only respectful, and truly helpful way to go. He said it like this:

> The result of psychotherapy can only be that the subject is, or is not, persuaded to feel, think, or act differently than has been his habit. The client changes some of his ways or he remains the same. The psychotherapist does not do anything but listen and talk. If there is any change in the client, it is, in the last analysis, brought about by the client himself. (1978, p. 190)

I want now to share one more piece that is relevant to the ironic cruelty discussed above that goes with acceptance of biopsychiatry's failure to meet the basic standards of scientific medicine in terms of objective standards of proof for its assertions. My experience is that maturity involves an ongoing, humbling process of disillusionment, a huge part of which involves repeated realizations that the teachings and beliefs of various personal and societal authorities are not worthy of the naïve trust that I had given them; of course, Szasz's lifework has been to disillusion us of trust in the beliefs and practices of psychiatry. In *The Myth of Psychotherapy*, Szasz provided interesting history about Sigmund Freud and Carl Jung. He highly values their work, and at the same time examines it in the light of these themes of autonomy and coercion. It is of note that he concluded his chapter on Jung with the assertion that Jung, despite his groundbreaking work on the secular cure of souls, exhibits the same failings as Freud in that "when the going gets difficult, Jung too falls back on regarding the mental patient as medically sick and the physician-psychotherapist as a medical healer." (p. 176)

As previously suggested, the identity of the counselor rests in a hierarchy of dependency on the psychiatrist. In my own work, I also discovered that this is perhaps most clearly seen when the going gets a bit tough. When counseling is not "working," when problems persist, especially those deemed severe as in "severe mental illness," counselors tend to defer to psychiatrists. We are already severely compromised when we refer to our clients as "patients." Such a designation obviously implies a medical model and a sick individual; worse, it reflects an attitude, a predisposition to respond in a medical way. Specifically, counselors readily and regularly refer their "patients" to psychiatrists for "medication," especially whenever the going gets a bit tough. This practice reflects a conscious, or at the very least an implicit deference and dependence on psychiatry, an acceptance of biopsychiatric theory and practice, especially when the going gets a bit tough, and a sad hopelessness and lack of confidence in both human nature and psychological theory and practice about the nature of distress and recovery. It reflects the deep conditioning of "mental health professionals," and the resultant demoralization best elucidated by psychologist Bruce Levine (2007). Worse still, such a conditioning also leads to our collaboration in the ongoing coercion and violations of liberty in the name of "therapy." Counselors refer people to psychiatrists and feel like they have done the right thing; like Pontius Pilate, their hands are now clean.

It seems to me that to sacrifice the reassuring notion that psychiatric coercion is help, or even further that a referral for drugs or electroshock is real help, may be handled in two ways. One of these is to harden the heart, to in fact become less compassionate. The other is to let the heart be broken, to directly face the deep grief and humility that comes with seeing another suffer and being unable to substantially help. Szasz often said that life is difficult and that tragedy is not uncommon; he faced it head on, and did his best to empower others in the only way he saw, which was to assume responsibility.

In a fairly recent interview, Szasz was asked what advice he might give to a potential counseling client. His response is a good segue to our next subject:

> My advice for a prospective client is to investigate his prospective therapist, to not trust him unless he proves himself trustworthy, and to be clear in his own mind about what he expects the therapist to do for him. Becoming a psychotherapy client is like becoming married: it may be a trap which it is much harder to escape from than to avoid. In short, beware of therapists, especially if you have reason to suspect that they will lock you up if they think you may kill yourself. (Howes, 2009)

Suicide

Like all counselors, I was taught the ethic that coercion in the cause of treating mental illness was a benevolent necessity, especially so with suicide. All counselor codes of ethics make clear that the ethical thing to do is to force treatment on anyone deemed to be actually suicidal, or even potentially suicidal if there is any doubt. As suicide is the main trigger for psychiatric coercion, and the primary justification for the shift from a voluntary counseling mode to a coercive treatment mode that inevitably means deprivation of liberty and forced administration of drugs, this is a pivotal point for any serious consideration of practicing Szasz. And it is a point that he took head on. In *Fatal Freedom* (1999) he deeply explores the subject. While psychiatry declares that suicide is a symptom of mental illness, Szasz insisted on defending human agency and wrote that it must be seen as a choice by a human agent; to do otherwise results in the annihilation of liberty and dignity. It is my view that anyone who avoids wrestling with the intellectual and moral terrain of the ethics of suicide cannot possibly be able to see, think and act clearly and consciously as a counselor. I will simply leave you with the title of Szasz's second book on the subject to summarize his judgment on the current practices in this area: *Suicide Prohibition: The Shame of Medicine* (2011).

The practical implications of Szasz's position on suicide are simple:

> Those who want to prevent a particular person from committing suicide must content themselves with their power, such as it might be, to persuade him to change his mind. (Szasz, 1992)

An obvious consequence of a counselor embracing mainstream ethics about suicide is that from a Szaszian perspective, whenever a suicidal dynamic comes forward, the counselor, no matter the outer title or appellation, immediately, and in my view tragically, shifts from counselor ally mode to potential jailer and adversary. Perhaps less obvious but equally true is that the counselor also once again forsakes his or her own beliefs and practices about counseling. As the going got tough, the counselor bailed out. There is of course no guarantee, but my own belief and experience is that in order to work through and recover from deep despair, emotional pain, and hopelessness about life, at least two things are often necessary, and both are forsaken when coercion comes into play. In my worldview, the paradox of change is that in order for something to change or transform at a deep level, it must first be faced and accepted for what it is. The paradox is that for suicidal despair to lessen it must be accepted and embraced. Psychiatry's refusal to accept such feelings, and to suppress them mightily, makes it difficult if not impossible to heal. A second related condition for lessening despair and restoring hope is the acceptance and listening to the despair and anguish by another person who is trusted. Conditions that encourage hiding or denying such feelings in order to avoid rejection or coercion are harmful and counterproductive; in my view it is absolutely necessary to reveal and share suicidal despair in order to get through it.

John Breeding, PhD

Chapter 9

CONCLUSION: A WAY OF BEING ETHICAL

Practicing Szasz is a way to be more ethical in a profession that is unethical in many ways. I use the term psychiatric oppression to refer to the ways that the mental health profession systematically mistreats those who are labeled mentally ill, and acts as an agency of social control for mainstream society. I want to end this paper by considering four primary mechanisms by which psychiatry enforces or holds other oppressions in place (Breeding, 2003). The first mechanism is suppression of thought and feeling. This is obvious in the use of psychoactive drugs and electroshock, and in overt coercion, less so with subtle threats, and labeling and paternalistic attitudes and practices. The work of Szasz is an ongoing denunciation of suppression of thought and behavior by psychiatry. In terms of counseling, Szasz emphasized relationships and, of course, autonomy and responsibility. While he clearly valued free expression, I think I place more emphasis on emotional release. Most importantly, Szasz wanted to empower individuals, and hated anything that put unnecessary constraints on personal freedom.

A second function of psychiatric oppression is distraction from social injustice by blaming the victim. I am not a pure libertarian like Szasz, but I am very clear that psychiatry blames and scapegoats individuals. In so doing, its primary function is political, and Szasz is by far the best source on dissecting and understanding the politics of psychiatric social control. His work is consistently about challenging oppression; the title of his book, *Liberation by Oppression* (2002), which compares slavery and psychiatry, is a good example of his direct assault on psychiatry's Orwellian function in our society. One major reason it is hard for people, and especially those who serve as agents of oppression, to delve deeply into Szasz's work is because he kills the sacred cow and forces one to see the slaughter for what it is. Jacob Sullum also asked Szasz whether he saw any encouraging developments since he started talking about psychiatric oppression. The answer reveals Szasz as a compassionate champion of the oppressed:

> The encouraging development is essentially the uprising of the slaves, the increasing protestation by ex-mental patients, many of whom call themselves victims. Through all kinds of groups, they have a voice now which they

> didn't have before. We should hear from the slaves. Psychiatry has always been described from the point of view of the psychiatrist; now the oppressed, the victim, the patient also has a voice. This I think is a very positive development. (Sullum, 2000)

My third point is that psychiatry enforces adherence to society's rules, however immoral and unethical they might be. Szasz laid out his game theory in his most famous book, *The Myth of Mental Illness* (1961), and he looked at the rules, at the games of life and of its institutions again and again. He believed in the value of politeness and etiquette, and of the necessity of the law to enforce order in the face of overt criminality, but his overarching value was liberty. Social psychology, most famously thought the works of Stanley Milgram (1975) on obedience and Philip Zimbardo (2008) on the power of the situation and social roles, has made clear that a relationship structure involving real or perceived differences in power is a setup for coercion. Subtle or not, these forces specifically pull us toward conformity and obedience to prescribed rules and behavior. Any counselor one who does not see this clearly will tend to consciously or unconsciously use their rank to control a client. A conscious decision for autonomy, and a vigilant guard against the situational pulls toward coercion are necessary to avoid becoming an adversary of that client. A key part of Szasz's solution was the contract between client and counselor, agreed to before the relationship begins. Knowing his work has definitely helped me in this regard.

Finally, psychiatry is oppressive by providing false hope and absolution, thus impeding or denying possible genuine movement toward greater freedom and autonomy. The hope one feels at getting help, at finding an explanation for the problem is tragically perverted when the explanation is that one is defective, and when the hope for a better life involves the use of drugs, much less electroshock, that may provide temporarily relief or suppression or stimulation, but lead to addiction, dependency and various long-term illnesses. Likewise the absolution may feel good—to believe that you are not to blame, your family is not to blame, society is not to blame, it is just regrettable that you suffer from "a chemical imbalance," "a lithium deficiency," "a brain defect" or some other unsubstantiated biological problem, but it is not your fault, and we can help you cope. This is a tragically false absolution, and as usual Szasz is best at striking at the heart of this lie. This false absolution utterly undermines the great values of freedom and liberty. Dependency on the identity of being a sick patient and dependency on the judgment of medical experts or any other kind of experts about one's life, together with dependency on drugs, destroys the movement toward greater autonomy and higher levels of personal responsibility. Thomas Szasz is not having any of this nonsense, and with his help neither am I.

References

Baughman, F. (2006). *The ADHD Fraud.* Trafford Publishing.

Baughman, F., & Breeding, J. (2003). "On Psychiatry and Child Protective Services in the United States." (http://www.wildestcolts.com/parenting/d-cps.html)

Breeding, J. (1998). "Drug Withdrawal and Emotional Recovery." *The Rights Tenet,* Winter 1998, National Association for Rights Protection and Advocacy. (May be read at www.wildestcolts.com/psych_opp/b-psychiatric_drugs/5-drug_wd.html).

Breeding, J. (2003). Press Release: Legislators Strike a Blow for Parent Rights: Two New Laws Put a Halt to Coercion of Parents to put Texas Children on Psychotropic Drugs. (http://www.wildestcolts.com/safe_ed/j-press_rel060403.html)

Breeding, J. (2003). *The Necessity Of Madness And Unproductivity: Psychiatric Oppression Or Human Transformation.* London: Chipmunka Press.

Breeding, J. (2006). "The Case of Sohrab Hassan: Assault on Liberty in the Texas Mental Health Courts." Journal of Humanistic Psychology, 46, 3, 2006, 243-254.

Breeding, J. (2007). *The Wildest Colts Make the Best Horses.* 3rd Edition. London: Chipmunka Publishing.

Breeding, J. (2009). *Coercion as cure: A critical history of psychiatry* by Thomas Szasz [Video review]. Retrieved from http://www.youtube.com/watch?v=khCdfL39Cos

Breeding, J. (2011) "Thomas Szasz: Philosopher of Liberty." *Journal of Humanistic Psychology*, 51, 1, 112-128.

Breeding, J. (2012) "A Psychiatric Assault on Liberty: The Case of Carolyn Barnes." (www.madinamerica.com/2012/12/a-psychiatric-assault-on-liberty-the-case-of-carolyn-barnes-2/)

Breggin, P. (1991). *Toxic Psychiatry.* New York: St. Martin's Press.

Burston, D. (2003). *Szasz, Laing, and existential psychotherapy.* Retrieved from http://www.ehinstitute.org/01-20-2004 (Accessed 4-20-10).

Citizens Commission on Human Rights International (1994). *Involuntary commitment*. Retrieved 12/31/2012, from http://www.cchrstl.org/documents/involuntary_commitment.pdf.)

Dexheimer, E. (10/20/2012). "State bills some court-detained mental patients for their care." *Austin American Statesman*. (http://www.statesman.com/news/news/state-regional/state-bills-some-court-detained-mental-patients-fo/nShyD/)

Dexheimer, E. (1/11/2013). "Attorney declared mentally fit to stand trial in shooting case." *Austin American Statesman*. (http://www.statesman.com/news/news/attorney-declared-mentally-fit-to-stand-trialnew-d/nTtL3/)

Duncan, B.L. & Miller, S.D. *The Heroic Client: Doing Client-Centered, Outcome-Informed Therapy*. San Francisco: Jossey-Bass.

Elias, M. (5/3/2007). "Mentally ill die 25 years earlier." *USA TODAY*.

Frank, L. R. (1978). *The History of Shock Treatment*. San Francisco.

Frank, L. R. (1998). *Random House Webster's Quotationary*. New York: Random House.

Frank, L. R. (2006). *The Electroshock Quotationary*. http://www.endofshock.com/102C_ECT.PDF).

Frank, L. R. (2008). *The electroshock quotationary*. Available at www.endofshock.com

Frank, L.R. (2011). *The Szasz Quotationary: The Wit and Wisdom of Thomas Szasz*. Kindle edition available at www.amazon.com.

Free Carolyn Barnes Blog (2012). http://freecarolynbarnes.blogspot.com.

Gatto, J. (2000). *The underground history of American education*. New York, NY: Oxford Village Press.

Gottstein, J. (2001). Legal Memorandum on the case of Rodney Yoder.
(http://gottsteinlaw.com/yoder/memo.pdf)

Hoch, P. (2004). Appendix: Documents from the Szasz affair at Upstate. In J. A. Schaler (Ed.), *Szasz under fire: The psychiatric abolitionist faces his critics* (pp. 393-402).Chicago, IL: Open Court. (Original work published 1962)
Hoeller, K. (Ed.). (1997). Thomas Szasz: Philosopher of psychiatry [Special issue]. *Review of Existential Psychology and Psychiatry, 23*(1-3).

Howes, R. (2009). "Seven Questions for Thomas Szasz," In *Therapy: A User's Guide to Psychotherapy* (*Psychology Today* blog).

Levine, B. (2007). *Surviving America's Depression Epidemic: How to Find morale,Energy, and Community in a world Gone Crazy.* White River Junction, Vermont: Chelsea Green Publishing Co.

Milgram, S. (1975). *Obedience to Authority.* NY: Harper & Row.

Schaler, J. A. (Ed.). (2004). *Szasz under fire: The psychiatric abolitionist faces his critics.* Chicago, IL: Open Court.

Slovenko, R. (2004). On Thomas Szasz, the meaning of mental illness, and the
therapeutic state: A critique. In J. A. Schaler (Ed.), *Szasz under fire: The psychiatricabolitionist faces his critics* (pp. 139-158). Chicago, IL: Open Court.

Scheff, T. (1984). *Being Mentally Ill: A Sociological Theory.* Aldine Publishing Co.

Sullum, J. (2000). Curing the Therapeutic State: Thoms Szasz Interviewed by Jacob Sullum. *Reason* magazine. (http://reason.com/archives/2000/07/01/curing-the-therapeutic-state-t)

Szasz, T. (1961). *The Myth of Mental Illness: Foundations of a Theory of personal Conduct.* New York: Hoeber-Harper.

Szasz, T. (1963). "Summary and Conclusions," *Law, Liberty, and Psychiatry: An Inquiry into the Social Uses of Mental Health Practices.* In L.R. Frank, *The Szasz*

Quotationary.

Szasz, T. (1963) *Law, Liberty, and Psychiatry: An Inquiry into the Social Uses of Mental Health Practices, ch. 4.* In L.R. Frank, *The Szasz Quotationary.*

Szasz, T. (1965). *Psychiatric Justice.* New York: Macmillan.

Szasz, T. (1965). *The Ethics of Psychoanalysis: The Theory and Method of Autonomous Psychotherapy.* New York: Basic Books, Inc.

Szasz, T. (1966) "Psychiatric Classification as a Strategy of Personal Constraint",
Ideology and Insanity: Essays on the Psychiatric Dehumanization of Man, ch. 12, sect. 6, 1970. In L.R. Frank, *The Szasz Quotationary.*

Szasz, T. (1970). *The manufacture of madness: A comparative study of the inquisition and the mental health movement.* Syracuse, NY: Syracuse University Press.

Szasz, T. (1970). *Ideology and Insanity: Essays on the Psychiatric Dehumanization of Man.* Garden City, NY: Doubleday Anchor.

Szasz, T. (1976). *Schizophrenia: The Sacred Symbol of Psychiatry.* New York: Basic Books, Inc.

Szasz, T. (1978). *The Myth of Psychotherapy: Mental Healing as Religion, Rhetoric and Repression.* Garden City, NY: Anchor Press.

Szasz, T. (1982). "On the Legitimacy of Psychiatric Power," *Metamedicine,* vol. 3. 1982. In L.R. Frank, *The Szasz Quotationary.*

Szasz, T. (1984). *The Therapeutic State: Psychiatry in the Mirror of Current Events.* Buffalo, NY: Prometheus Books.

Szasz, T. (1987). *Insanity: The Idea and Its Consequences.* New York: John Wiley.

Szasz, T. (1992). "The Fatal Temptation: Drug Control and Suicide." *The Medicalization of Everyday Life: Selected Essays,* ch. 11, sect. 1, 2007. In L.R. Frank, *The Szasz Quotationary.*

Szasz, T. (1993) *A Lexicon of Lunacy: Metaphoric Malady,Moral Responsibility, and Psychiatry*. New Brunswick, New Jersey: Transaction Publishers.

Szasz, T. (1993). "Foreword" to Seth Farber, *Madness, Heresy, and the Rumor of Angels:The Revolt Against the Mental Health System*.

Szasz, T. (1994). *Cruel Compassion: Psychiatric Control of Society's Unwanted*. New York: John Wiley.

Szasz, T. (1997). *The Manufacture of Madness: A Comparative Study of the Inquisition and the Mental Health Movement*. Syracuse University Press.

Szasz, T. (1997). Mental illness is still a myth. *Review of Existential Psychology and Psychiatry, 23*, 70-80.

Szasz, T. (1999). *Fatal freedom: The ethics and politics of suicide*. Westport, CT:
Praeger.

Szasz, T. (2002). *Liberation by oppression: A comparative study of slavery and psychiatry*. New Brunswick, NJ: Transaction Books.

Szasz, T. (2004a). An autobiographical sketch. J. A. Schaler (Ed.), *Szasz under fire: The psychiatric abolitionist faces his critics* (pp. 1-28). Chicago, IL: Open Court.

Szasz, T. (2004b). Politeness. In *Words to the wise: A medical-philosophical dictionary*. New Brunswick, NJ: Transaction.

Szasz, T. (2004c). Reply to Kendell. In J. A. Schaler (Ed.), *Szasz under fire: The psychiatric abolitionist faces his critics* (pp. 49-56). Chicago, IL: Open Court.

Szasz, T. (2004d). Reply to Simon. In J. A. Schaler (Ed.), *Szasz under fire: The psychiatric abolitionist faces his critics* (pp. 202-224). Chicago, IL: Open Court.

Szasz, T. (2004e). Reply to Slovenko. In J. A. Schaler (Ed.), *Szasz under fire: The psychiatric abolitionist faces his critics* (pp. 159-178). Chicago, IL: Open Court.

Szasz, T. (2007) *Coercion as Cure: A Critical History of Psychiatry.* New Brunswick,NJ: Transaction Publishers.

Szasz, T. (2008a). Debunking antipsychiatry: Laing, law, and largactil. *Existential Analysis, 19*(2), 316-343.

Szasz, T. (2008b). Speech at Citizens Commission on Human Rights Event. (https://www.youtube.com/watch?v=zQegsqYhuZE).

Szasz, T. (2011). *Suicide Prohibition: The Shame of Medicine.* Syracuse University Press.

Whitaker, R. (2010). Anatomy *of an Epidemic: Magic Bullets, Psychiatric Drugs, and the Astonishing Rise of Mental Illness in America.* New York: Crown Publishers. Wikipedia. (2010). Ignaz Semmelweis. Retrieved from http://en.wikipedia.org/wiki/Ignaz_Semmelweis.

Wyatt, R. (2000). *An interview with Thomas Szasz, MD: Liberty & the practice of psychotherapy.* Retrieved from http://www.psychotherapy.net/interview/Thomas_Szasz

Zimbardo, P. (2008). *The Lucifer Effect: Understanding How Good People Turn Evil.* NY: Random House.

Appendix

The Wisdom and Wit of Thomas Szasz: Selected Quotations

Leonard Roy Frank, editor

John Breeding, PhD

Introduction

With the publication of *The Myth of Mental Illness* in 1961, Thomas Szasz became the center of a heated controversy. A psychiatrist himself, he rejected the foundational beliefs of his profession, contending in effect that psychiatrists are fake doctors who use fake treatments to "cure" the fake diseases of fake patients. His colleagues countered with arguments and personal attacks that failed to offset the impact Szasz's views had on public opinion at the time. Widespread coverage in professional publications and the mainstream media soon made Szasz the most controversial figure in contemporary psychiatry and a serious threat to the prestige and power of the profession.

Recognizing the danger the Szaszian perspective represented, his colleagues decided on a new tack: they adopted a policy of *Totschweigetaktik*, the German word for "death by silence," wherein fresh ideas and approaches are ignored rather than challenged, in the belief that they will die for lack of "the oxygen of attention." It was a shrewd tactic. Despite a continuous flow of writings during the 60 years since then (more than 30 books and 800 articles), Szasz has practically disappeared from the public's awareness while organized psychiatry has grown in popularity to the point that it is now perhaps the world's major secular belief system.

Why the strong reaction? Because the implications of Szasz's views on psychiatry and its role in society are huge. Were they widely accepted, the entire psychiatric system, built as it is on fraud, fear, and force, might fall like a house of cards.

With its dynamic and thought-provoking ideas, my hope is that this selection of Szasz's quotes will help awaken people to the menace psychiatry poses to a free society and motivate them to take direct political action to reverse the slide to what Szasz names and describes as "the therapeutic state, whose aim is not to provide favorable conditions for life, liberty, and the pursuit of happiness, but to repair the defective mental health of its citizens."

All the quotations in the appendix are drawn from *The Szasz Quotationary*, which I edited with Szasz's cooperation. Together we co-published it as an e-book in 2012.

Throughout this selection, and the *TSQ* as well, Szasz uses terms like *mental illness, psychiatric diagnosis, mental hospital,* and *psychiatric treatment* while rejecting their conventional meanings. To avoid defacing the text, he has largely refrained from putting such expressions between quotation marks each time they appear.

A minority of Szasz's quotations differ in substance or style from the original writings, which are referenced with each entry. Szasz made or approved all such changes.

Leonard Roy Frank
San Francisco

Section 1

LIBERTY AND RESPONSIBILITY

A person should be deprived of liberty only if proved guilty of breaking the law.

"Summary and Conclusions," *Law, Liberty, and Psychiatry: An Inquiry into the Social Uses of Mental Health Practices,* 1963.

An individual is the end product of the decisions he has made. He who fails to make decisions, for the consequences of which he is responsible, is not a fully realized person. The ego, the self, the personality — call it what you will — comes into being and grows through the process of making responsible decisions.

"Epilogue," *Law, Liberty, and Psychiatry: An Inquiry into the Social Uses of Mental Health Practices,* 1963.

Autonomy is a positive concept. It is freedom to develop one's self — to increase one's knowledge, improve one's skills, and achieve responsibility for one's conduct. And it is freedom to lead one's own life, to choose among alternative courses of action so long as no injury to others results.

The Ethics of Psychoanalysis: The Theory and Method of Autonomous Psychotherapy, ch. 1, 1965.

All history teaches us, those who would take from man his moral burdens — be they priests or warlords, politicians or psychiatrists — must also take from him his liberty and hence his very humanity.

"Mental Illness Is a Myth," *New York Times Magazine,* 12 June 1966.

The crucial moral characteristic of the human condition is the dual experience of freedom of the will and personal responsibility. Since freedom and responsibility are two aspects of the same phenomenon, they invite comparison with the proverbial knife that cuts both ways. One of its edges implies options: we call it freedom. The other edge implies obligations: we call it responsibility.

"Introduction," *The Theology of Medicine: The Political-Philosophical Foundations of Medical Ethics,* 1977.

I favor free trade in drugs for the same reason the Founders favored free trade in ideas: in a free society it is none of the government's business what ideas a man puts into his mind;

85

likewise, it should be none of its business what drug he puts into his body.

"Drug Prohibition" (1978), *The Therapeutic State: Psychiatry in the Mirror of Current Events,* 1984.

In a society dedicated to individual freedom and responsibility, self-injurious behavior cannot justify loss of liberty. The state, the family, and the medical profession must restrict themselves to offering help; they must eschew forcing help on unwilling persons and, indeed, ought to be prevented by law from doing so. Granted, some of the increase in liberty so gained might be purchased at the cost of the impaired health, or even death, of some persons who make themselves ill or who want to kill themselves; but freedom must entail the right to make the "wrong" choices.

"A Critical Look at Psychiatry" (1980), *The Therapeutic State: Psychiatry in the Mirror of Current Events,* p. 30, 1984.

Freedom of belief lies at the heart of individual liberty and dignity. That is why I maintain that "deluded" patients are as entitled to their beliefs as "enlightened" psychiatrists are to theirs. Like clergy of different faiths, or believers and unbelievers, each should be protected from being coerced by the other.

"Law and Psychiatry: The Problems That Will Not Go Away," *Journal of Mind and Behavior,* Summer and Autumn, 1990.

When a man says he is Jesus or makes some other claim that seems to us outrageous, we call him psychotic and lock him up in a madhouse. Freedom of speech is only for normal people.

"Schizophrenia," *The Untamed Tongue: A Dissenting Dictionary,* 1990.

People are free in proportion as the State protects them from *others;* and are oppressed in proportion as the State protects them from *themselves.*

"Therapeutic State," *The Untamed Tongue: A Dissenting Dictionary,* 1990.

Section 2

PSYCHIATRY

Psychiatry is much more intimately related to ethics than it is to medicine. I use the word "psychiatry" here to refer to the contemporary discipline concerned with problems in living, not with diseases of the brain, which belong to neurology.

"The Myth of Mental Illness" (1960), *Ideology and Insanity: Essays on the Psychiatric Dehumanization of Man,* ch. 2, sect. 1, 1970.

There are, and can be, no abuses of institutional psychiatry, because institutional psychiatry is, itself, an abuse; similarly, there were, and could be, no abuses of the Inquisition because the Inquisition was, itself, an abuse. Indeed, just as the Inquisition was the characteristic abuse of Christianity, so institutional psychiatry is the characteristic abuse of medicine.

"Introduction," *The Manufacture of Madness: A Comparative Study of the Inquisition and the Mental Health Movement,* 1970.

Institutional Psychiatry is a continuation of the Inquisition. All that has changed is the vocabulary and the social style.

The Manufacture of Madness: A Comparative Study of the Inquisition and the Mental Health Movement, ch. 1, 1970.

The principle social institutions involved in the theory and practice of psychiatric violence are the State, the family, and the medical profession. The State authorizes the involuntary incarceration of "dangerous" mental patients; the family approves and makes use of the arrangement; and the medical profession, through psychiatry, administers the institution and supplies the necessary justifications for it.

The Manufacture of Madness: A Comparative Study of the Inquisition and the Mental Health Movement, ch. 15, 1970.

We don't deny that there's a Church of Rome that propagates a faith called Catholicism; or that there's a Church of England that propagates a faith called Anglicanism. But we deny that there's a Church of America — better known as the National Institute of Mental Health — that propagates a faith called Psychiatry. The Church of America would have us believe that we can lead lives of ambition without anxiety; that we can have success without strife, sociability without conflict, reward without punishment, and

pleasure without pain. All this and heaven, too, is the promise, if only we have faith in Psychiatry.
October 1971
"In the Church of America, Psychiatrists Are Priests," *Hospital Physician,* October 1971.

"Superstition is to religion," wrote Voltaire, "what astrology is to astronomy...." Just so is psychiatry to medicine.
"Psychiatry," *The Untamed Tongue: A Dissenting Dictionary,* 1990.

There are two kinds of psychiatry: voluntary (contractual) and involuntary (institutional). To confuse them is like confusing ally and adversary, freedom and slavery.
"Psychiatry," *The Untamed Tongue: A Dissenting Dictionary,* 1990.

In science, it's dangerous to lie: if discovered, the liar is cast out of the group as a faker and fraud. In religion, politics, and psychiatry, it's dangerous to tell the truth: if discovered, the truth-teller is cast out of the group as a heretic or a traitor.
"Social Relations," *The Untamed Tongue: A Dissenting Dictionary,* 1990.

The primary purpose of psychiatry is not medical-therapeutic because its historical mandate and primary purpose is not to remedy a patient's diseases but to soothe society's conscience about its deplorable behavior toward unwanted persons.
"Remembering Krafft-Ebing," *Ideas on Liberty,* January 2000.

As long as we have no historical-moral accounting and hence no collective memory for psychiatry's crimes against humanity — similar to the accounting and memory for the wrongs of Christianity recognized by the papacy, slavery recognized by the American people, and the Holocaust recognized by Germany and the Western world — no *ad hoc* criticism of psychiatric "abuses" will have any impact on the prestige and power of psychiatry and no criticism of the concept of mental illness will be persuasive.
Pharmacracy: Medicine and Politics in America, ch. 5, 2001.

Psychiatry is the single most important weapon in the modern state's war against individual liberty and personal responsibility.
Faith in Freedom: Libertarian Principles and Psychiatric Practices, ch. 11, 2004.

Once you use the language of psychiatry, you have already capitulated. There is no mental illness. There is no psychiatric diagnosis. These is no psychiatric treatment. These are just words used by more powerful people against less powerful people in the name of helping them but actually to control them or to punish them or both.

Lew Rockwell Internet interview, *The Lew Rockwell Show,* 20 November 2008.

Modern psychiatry — with its *Diagnosis and Statistical Manuals* of nonexisting diseases and their coercive cures — is a monument to quackery on a scale undreamed of in the annals of medicine.
Psychiatry: The Science of Lies, ch. 1, 2008.

Section 3

MENTAL ILLNESS

Mental illness is a myth, whose function is to disguise and thus render more palatable the bitter pill of moral conflicts in human relations.

"The Myth of Mental Illness" (1960), *Ideology and Insanity: Essays on the Psychiatric Dehumanization of Man,* ch. 2, sect. 7, 1970.

In contemporary America [mental health] has come to mean conformity to the demands of society. According to the commonsense definition, mental health is the ability to play the game of social living, and to play it well. Conversely, mental illness is the refusal to play, or the inability to play well.

Law, Liberty, and Psychiatry: An Inquiry into the Social Uses of Mental Health Practices, ch. 17, 1963.

The actual, though covert, aim of psychiatric classification is to degrade and socially segregate the individual identified as a mental patient, thereby creating a class of justifiably persecuted scapegoats.

"Whither Psychiatry?" (1966), *Ideology and Insanity: Essays on the Psychiatric Dehumanization of Man,* ch. 13, sect. 9, 1970.

In vain does the alleged madman insist that he is not sick; his inability to "recognize" that he is, is regarded as a hallmark of his illness. In vain does he reject treatment and hospitalization as forms of torture and imprisonment; his refusal to submit to psychiatric authority is regarded as a further sign of his illness.

"Preface," *The Manufacture of Madness: A Comparative Study of the Inquisition and the Mental Health Movement,* 1970.

Bodily illness stands in the same relation to mental illness as a defective television set stands to a bad television program. Of course, the word "sick" is often used metaphorically. We call jokes "sick," economies "sick," sometimes even the whole world "sick"; but only when we call minds "sick" do we systematically mistake and strategically misinterpret metaphor for fact — and send for the doctor to "cure" the "illness." It is as if a television viewer were to send for a television repairman because he dislikes the program he sees on the screen.

"Preface to the Second Edition," *The Myth of Mental Illness:*

91

Foundations of a Theory of Personal Conduct, rev. ed., 1974 (1961).

In the Age of Faith, men and women had to, and wanted to, call their spiritual problems sins and their spiritual authorities fathers, who, in turn, called them children. In the Age of Medicine, men and women have to, and want to, call their spiritual problems sicknesses and their spiritual authorities doctors, who, in turn, call them patients.
"The Metaphors of Faith and Folly" (1975), *The Theology of Medicine: The Political-Philosophical Foundations of Medical Ethics,* 1977.

Delusion: a belief said to be false by someone who does not share it.
"Mental Illness," *Heresies,* 1976.

If a man claims that the pope is infallible, he is a pious Catholic; if he claims that he himself is infallible, he is a paranoid schizophrenic.
"Schizophrenia," *Heresies,* 1976.

The belief that schizophrenia is a brain disease conceals moral and social problems not susceptible to solution by medical research or treatment.
"Schizophrenia," *The Untamed Tongue: A Dissenting Dictionary,* 1990.

The notion that there is no schizophrenia is so unpalatable — its implications are so devastating — that the authorities cannot deign to acknowledge it, even as a possibility. If there were no schizophrenia, there would be no medical, psychiatric, public health, or therapeutic justification for arresting, imprisoning, and involuntarily drugging people we call schizophrenics. There would be no civil commitment and no insanity defense.
Where would that leave us?
Appendix I, *Liberation by Oppression: A Comparative Study of Slavery and Psychiatry,* 2002.

Mental illness is an oxymoron whose function is to deceive others and oneself.
Psychiatry: The Science of Lies, ch. 4, sect. 4, 2008.

Section 4

PSYCHIATRIC INTERVENTIONS

Institutional psychiatry enforces role conformity by defining role deviance as mental illness punishable by commitment.

"The Insanity Plea and the Insanity Verdict" (1967), *Ideology and Insanity: Essays on the Psychiatric Dehumanization of Man,* ch. 8, sect. 3, 1970.

The mental patient, we say, *may be* dangerous: he may harm himself or someone else. But we, society, *are* dangerous: we rob him of his good name and of his liberty, and subject him to tortures called "treatments."

The Manufacture of Madness: A Comparative Study of the Inquisition and the Mental Health Movement, ch. 15, 1970.

Whereas in the Age of Faith, to lose one's faith, or to repudiate its object, God, meant the loss of one's humanity and resulted in the expulsion from the social order of the offending individual as a heretic — so, in the Age of Reason, to lose one's reason, or to repudiate its object, Reality, means the loss of one's humanity and results in the expulsion from the social order of the offending individual as a madman. Who, then, could scoff at, much less oppose, God in a Theological Society? Only a heretic! And who can scoff at, much less oppose mental health in a Therapeutic Society? Only a madman! No punishment could be unjust, no therapy can be unjustified, in society's efforts to combat these threats to its core values.

"Introduction," *The Age of Madness: The History of Involuntary Mental Hospitalization Presented in Selected Texts,* 1973.

There is no medical, moral, or legal justification for involuntary psychiatric interventions. They are crimes against humanity.

"Summary" (sect. 10), *The Myth of Mental Illness: Foundations of a Theory of Personal Conduct,* rev. ed., 1974 (1961).

Formerly, when priests ruled and people exalted the spirit, the favorite methods of punishments were breaking men's bodies on the rack and the wheel. Today, when physicians rule and people exalt the body, our favorite punishments are breaking men's minds with drugs, electrical convulsions, and surgical amputations of the brain.

"Punishment," *Heresies,* 1976.

Coerced psychiatric personality change — even (or especially) if it entails "helping" a person to give up his "psychotic delusions" — closely resembles coerced religious conversion.
Psychiatric Slavery, ch. 8, sect. 1, 1977.

Commitment, involuntary mental hospitalization, is, of course, the paradigm of psychiatric power. In my opinion, it is also a paradigm of the perversion of power: for if the "patient" is not a criminal, then he or she has a right to liberty; and if the patient is a criminal, then he or she ought to be restrained and punished by the criminal law, like anyone else....
Involuntary mental hospitalization and the insanity defense should be seen for what they are: symmetrical symbols of psychiatric power. In the one case, the psychiatrist "accuses" the innocent; in the other, he "excuses" the guilty. Civil commitment and the insanity defense both create and confirm the impression of psychiatric expertise, where none exists. Civil commitment and the insanity defense also foster the impression that they provide a socially beneficial solution for troubling problems of human existence, when, actually both aggravate these problems. In short, both are inimical to, and indeed incompatible with, the principles of a free society.
"On the Legitimacy of Psychiatric Power," *Metamedicine,* vol. 3, 1982.

It is stupid to speak of "involuntary psychiatric treatments" when what we mean are psychiatrically rationalized assaults.
"Psychiatry," *The Untamed Tongue: A Dissenting Dictionary,* 1990.

The psychiatric profession's most distinguishing feature is the deliberate, systematic dehumanization of man, in the name of mental health.
"Forward" to Seth Farber, *Madness, Heresy, and the Rumor of Angels: The Revolt Against the Mental Health System,* 1993.

Psychiatrists now attribute resistance to psychiatric coercion to "anosognosia," an alleged brain disease. Priests hunting heretics were more modest: they were satisfied with destroying their adversaries' bodies by burning them at the stake. Psychiatrists have higher aspirations: true soul murderers, they deny their adversaries' capacity to possess moral agency. Mental patients who refuse psychiatric drugs do so because they suffer from anosognosia — "a lack of awareness of mental illness... common among patients with schizophrenia who are nonadherent to antipsychotics."

Antipsychiatry: Quackery Squared, ch. 1, sect. 5, 2009. The quoted passage is from Olfson, M., et al., "Awareness of Illness and Nonadherence to Antipsychotic Medications among Persons with Schizophrenia," *Psychiatric Services,* February 2006.

Psychiatric abuses — epitomized first by forced hospitalization and now by forced drugging — are driven by a combination of sadism, grandiosity, naiveté, and venality. Today, pharmaceutical companies in effect bribe psychiatrists to administer psychoactive drugs to as many people as possible and write glowing reports about the drug's therapeutic effectiveness and lack of side effects.

Coercion as Cure: A Critical History of Psychiatry, ch. 4, sect. 1, 2007.

Murdering mental patients, which doctors in National Socialist Germany called "euthanasia" and "mercy death," is the most extreme form of psychiatric treatment. Mutilating the healthy brains of mental patients — which doctors first called "prefrontal lobotomy" and now call "psychosurgical treatment" — is a close second. With good reason Walter Freeman, the most notorious lobotomist in history, is often compared to Josef Mengele, the emblem of Nazi medical criminality.

Coercion as Cure: A Critical History of Psychiatry, ch. 6, sect. 1, 2007.

The central issue facing psychiatry and our society today is not whether a particular psychiatric intervention works or does not, whether it helps or harms the patient, whether it is therapeutic or toxic, whether it prevents suicide or promotes it. The central issue is whether contact between psychiatrist and patient is voluntary or involuntary, consensual or coercive. All other issues are secondary.

"Conclusion" (sect. 2), *Coercion as Cure: A Critical History of Psychiatry,* 2007.

Psychiatric coercion is medicalized terrorism.

"Psychiatry: The Shame of Medicine," *The Freeman: Ideas on Liberty,* March 2009.

John Breeding, PhD

Section 5

PSYCHIATRISTS

For the most part, psychiatrists are engaged in attempts to change the behavior and values of individuals, groups, institutions, and sometimes even of nations. Hence, psychiatry is a form of social engineering. It should be recognized as such.

"Preface," *Law, Liberty, and Psychiatry: An Inquiry into the Social Uses of Mental Health Practices,* 1963.

The fundamental parallel between master and slave on the one hand, and institutional psychiatrist and involuntarily hospitalized patient on the other, lies in this: in each instance, the former member of the pair defines the social role of the latter, and casts him in that role by force.

"Involuntary Mental Hospitalization: A Crime Against Humanity" (1968), *Ideology and Insanity: Essays on the Psychiatric Dehumanization of Man,* ch. 9, sect. 5, 1970.

Psychiatric training, above all else, is the ritualized indoctrination of the young physician into the theory and practice of psychiatric violence.

"Psychiatry," *The Second Sin,* 1973.

Therapeutism: successor to patriotism. The last refuge — or the first, depending on the authority consulted — of scoundrels. The creed that justifies proclaiming undying love for those we hate, and inflicting merciless punishment on them in the name of treating them for diseases whose principal symptoms are their refusal to submit to our domination.

"Therapeutic State," *The Second Sin,* 1973.

Psychiatrists realize that their entire enterprise hinges on society's acceptance of the proposition that human beings diagnosed as mentally ill have a brain disease that deprives them of free will.

"Introduction," *A Lexicon of Lunacy: Metaphoric Malady, Moral Responsibility, and Psychiatry,* 1993.

Ever since I was an adolescent, when I set my sights on going to medical school, I had believed that the physician's role is to help relieve the suffering of individuals who ask for and accept his help, and that the psychiatrist is committing a grave moral wrong if he imprisons individuals who neither seek nor want his help.

"An Autobiographical Sketch" (sect. 7), in Schaler, J. A., ed., *Szasz Under Fire: The Psychiatric Abolitionist Faces His Critics,* 2004.

Psychiatrists are in a hopeless fix. They cannot become honest professionals so long as they pretend to be physicians diagnosing and treating mental diseases. Yet they cannot acknowledge that they are advocates and adversaries in human conflicts and curers of souls in distress, lest they lose their credibility and status as medical doctors.

"Psychiatry," *Words to the Wise: A Medical-Philosophical Dictionary,* 2004.

Section 6

PSYCHOANALYSIS

Beware of the psychoanalyst who analyzes jokes rather than laughs at them.
"Psychoanalysis," *The Second Sin,* 1973.

Freud was an ambitious and slick operator, a "mental healer" on the make among the famous, the rich, and the gullible.
"The Pretensions of the Freudian Cult," *The Spectator,* 5 October 1985.

Psychoanalysis is a religion disguised as a science. As Abraham received the Laws of God from Jehovah to whom he claimed to have had special access, so Freud received the Laws of Psychology from the Unconscious to which he claimed to have had special access.
"Psychoanalysis," *The Untamed Tongue: A Dissenting Dictionary,* 1990.

Psychoanalysis is a pseudomedical cult.
"The Religion Called 'Psychiatry'" (1987), *A Lexicon of Lunacy: Metaphoric Malady, Moral Responsibility, and Psychiatry,* ch. 5, 1993.

Psychoanalytic treatment stands in the same relation to ordinary conversation as the Eucharist wafer stands in the relation to a cracker.
"Psychiatry," *Words to the Wise: A Medical-Philosophical Dictionary,* 2004.

Although Freud liked to claim that he had disturbed the sleep of mankind, the opposite is the case: he provided people with the comforts of a false explanation.
Psychiatry: The Science of Lies, ch. 2, sect. 2, 2008.

Section 7

PSYCHOTHERAPY

The purpose of autonomous psychotherapy is to aid the client in his efforts to live more effectively according to his own goals, both present and future. This does not mean that the client's moral conceptions and conduct remain unscrutinized. On the contrary, such scrutiny is an essential part of therapy. The point I wish to emphasize is that the therapist is contractually and morally committed to avoid influencing his client by any means other than by conversation with him. Thus, the psychotherapist may not speak about the client to others (not even to colleagues), testify for or against him in a court of law, or hospitalize or medically treat the client with or without his consent.

Law, Liberty, and Psychiatry: An Inquiry into the Social Uses of Mental Health Practices, ch. 16, 1963.

Many modern psychotherapists have adopted, as their credo, Socrates' declaration that "unexamined life is not worth living." But for modern man this is not enough. We should pledge ourselves to the proposition that the irresponsible life is not worth living.

"Epilogue," *Law, Liberty, and Psychiatry: An Inquiry into the Social Uses of Mental Health Practices,* 1963. The quoted passage is from Plato, *Apology,* sect. 38, 4th cent. B.C.E.

The ethic of the psychotherapeutic relationship is communicated by what actually occurs between psychotherapist and client. What distinguishes this enterprise from others is that, although the therapist tries to help his client, he does not "take care of him." The client takes care of himself. Furthermore, the client realizes that he is "expected to recover," not in any medical or psychopathological sense, but in a purely moral sense, by learning more about himself and by assuming greater responsibility for his conduct. He learns that only self-knowledge and responsible commitment and action can set him free. In sum, autonomous psychotherapy is an actual small-scale demonstration of the nature and feasibility of the ethic of autonomy in human relationships.

The Ethics of Psychoanalysis: The Theory and Method of Autonomous Psychotherapy, ch. 1, 1965.

People seeking help from psychotherapists can be divided into two groups: those who wish to confront their difficulties and shortcomings and change their lives by changing themselves; and those who wish to avoid the inevitable consequences of their life strategies through the magical or tactical intervention of the therapist in their lives.

"Psychotherapy," *The Second Sin,* 1973.

The autonomous psychotherapist's role vis-à-vis his client is like the court jester's vis-à-vis the monarch: the therapist confronts the client with painful reality, but in as friendly a way as possible; the client retains complete control over how, if at all, he uses what the therapist tells him.

"Psychotherapy," *The Second Sin,* 1973.

The therapist's initial task is to create a context of comfort, safety, and trust in the therapeutic situation, enabling the client to feel in control, especially about beginning and ending the relationship.

Ryan Howes interview, "Seven Questions for Thomas Szasz," *In Therapy: A User's Guide to Psychotherapy* (*Psychology Today* blog), 28 January 2009.

Section 8

MISCELLANIES

Achieving dignity and individuality is always a personal affair. It can be facilitated or hindered; but, in the end, each person must do it for himself.

"Epilogue," *Law, Liberty, and Psychiatry: An Inquiry into the Social Uses of Mental Health Practices,* 1963.

The fundamental conflicts in human life are not between competing ideas — one "true" and the other "false" — but rather between those who hold power and use it to oppress others, and those who are oppressed by power and seek to free themselves from it.

The Manufacture of Madness: A Comparative Study of the Inquisition and the Mental Health Movement, ch. 4, 1970.

To grow up, one must learn to take oneself seriously, to take life seriously, and to take others seriously. This is a simple thing to say but is, actually, a terrifyingly hard thing to achieve. It is especially difficult to achieve for a child whose parents do not take him seriously; that is, who do not expect proper behavior from him, do not discipline him, and, finally, do not respect him enough to tell him the truth.

"Tragic Failures," *National Review,* 26 May 1972.

Marx said that religion was the opiate of the people. In the United States today, opiates are the religion of the people.

"Drugs," *The Second Sin,* 1973.

Self-respect is to the soul as oxygen is to the body. Deprive a person of oxygen, and you kill his body; deprive him of self-respect, and you kill his spirit.

"Social Relations," *The Second Sin,* 1973.

Power corrupts. But so does powerlessness. Respect for human dignity requires a wide distribution of power.... Limited power is thus a necessary, but not a sufficient, condition for the flowering of respect for self and others. The additional requirement for it is the love of justice.

"Social Relations," *The Second Sin,* 1973.

A spirited engine is a good engine, a spirited horse is a good horse, and a spirited man is a good man — but a spirited woman is a

"masculine" woman. This is how the language of male chauvinism refracts "reality."
"Men and Women," *Heresies,* 1976.

As the base rhetorician uses language to increase his own power, to produce converts to his own cause, and to create loyal followers of his own person, so the noble rhetorician uses language to wean men from their inclination to depend on authority, to encourage them to think and speak clearly, and to teach them to be their own masters.
The Myth of Psychotherapy: Mental Healing as Religion, Rhetoric, and Repression, ch. 2, sect. 4, 1978.

Student: What is the single most important quality of a person?
Szasz: Courage [*pause*].... Courage to be subversive.
Exchange, quoted in James A. Prevost, "Remarks of a Student," *Asclepius at Syracuse: Thomas Szasz, Libertarian Humanist* (Proceedings), vol. 1, p. 8, 1980.

There are two kinds of "disabled" persons: Those who dwell on what they have lost and those who concentrate on what they have left.
"Personal Conduct," *The Untamed Tongue: A Dissenting Dictionary,* 1990.

What is a friend? For some, a sycophant; for others, an incorruptible but loving critic.
"Social Relations," *The Untamed Tongue: A Dissenting Dictionary,* 1990.

Man's reach for doing the right thing has always exceeded his grasp. Perhaps therein lies the engine of moral progress.
Faith in Freedom: Libertarian Principles and Psychiatric Practices, ch. 2, 2004.

History is a chronicle of people clinging to erroneous ideas authenticated as religious or scientific truths.
"On Not Admitting Error," *The Freeman: Ideas on Liberty,* March 2007.